EVOLUTION OF YOGA

...Discusses cogently how to lead our lives usefully by remaining connected with Mother Nature. It explains lucidly the principles of yoga, yogic exercises to be performed for keeping different parts of the body healthy and free of disease, the yogic diet and how it can be modified according to the present day and age, ways of keeping the mind relaxed and means to connect the mind with the body on the one hand and with the soul on the other.

EVOLUTION OF YOGA

DR. BHARAT BHUSHAN SAHI

M.B.B.S.,M.S.,D.O.(London)

New Age Books

ISBN: 978-81-7822-317-9
First Edition: Delhi, 2009

Published by
NEW AGE BOOKS
A-44 Naraina Industrial Area Phase-I
New Delhi 110028 (India)
Email: nab@vsnl.in
Website: www.newagebooksindia.com

Printed in India
at Shri Jainendra Press
A-45 Naraina Phase-I, New Delhi-110028

PREFACE

Industrialization after the Second World War has made the world a prosperous place to live in. Prosperity can be seen in every sphere of life: in higher standard of living, transportation, food, communication, education, etc.

People have started eating convenience foods, readily available cooked foods, frozen foods, packed foods, tinned foods, etc. These foods not only lack freshness, but most of their nutritional ingredients are destroyed in the process of cooking, freezing and preserving them. They are far less nourishing than fresh ones.

Transportation such as cars, motorcycles, buses, etc. have made people lethargic and less active. It is essential that toxic energy (energy containing waste products) is eliminated from the body and is replaced with fresh vital energy. If energy is not used up, energy saturated with toxic products is accumulated in the body causing different ailments. Constant accumulation of toxic energy in the body leads to chronic diseases such as heart disease, high blood pressure, diabetes, arthritis, chronic indigestion, etc. Over eating manifests in the form of obesity, which leads to so many other ailments.

The high pace of life has given rise to increased desires for gratification and more stress. To fulfill those desires, more resources are required which leads to a vicious cycle.

To release stress and satisfy the senses people turn to over eating, drinking alcohol, excessive tea or coffee and become addicted to various stimulants classified as drugs.

To solve this problem, scientists and sociologists have turned their attention towards our ancestors, their ways of living, their eating habits and how they used to spend their leisure time. Their attention was drawn towards yoga, because our ancestors used to lead their lives based on principles of yoga, which teaches us how to spend our lives constructively by remaining connected to our mother energy (God). A yogi lives life in harmony with the principles of Mother Nature.

This book is written to explore and explain how to spend our lives usefully by remaining connected with the Supreme (Nature) by following yogic principles.

I have made an effort to explain the principles of yoga, the yogic exercises to be performed for keeping different parts of the body healthy and free of disease, the yogic diet and how this diet can be modified according to the present day and age, ways of keeping the mind relaxed and means to connect the mind with the body on the one hand and with the soul on the other.

I am confident readers will enjoy reading this book, which I have divided into short chapters. I hope it allows them to understand ways to adopt a healthier, wiser and more constructive lifestyle.

ACKNOWLEDGEMENTS

This book is being brought to you entirely due to my own efforts, except for the help of my publisher in editing and formatting.

Although my interest in the subject of yoga dates back to childhood because of family traditions, but the idea of writing this book would not have originated if I had not joined Yoga group at Asoka Park, New Friends Colony, New Delhi, India, Fourteen years ago after my early retirement. This group has been in existence for over 25 years, which very much proves that traditional yoga has been practised in small groups, ever since it was invented. In the group Mr. Verinder Mehta acted as my mentor and practical learning of Yoga Asanas and pranayam I learnt from him. Mr. Mehta had to leave three years ago to spread the cause of yoga to a wider city audience and the reins were taken over by Mr. Mohinder Singh, an advocate. I wish to thank all the colleagues in the group, but my special thanks to Mr. Mehta and Mr. Mohinder Singh for their guidance.

Contents

INTRODUCTION

Talk of yoga and people start thinking about different postural exercises called *Yog Asanas*. Actually yoga is a way of life based on certain principles to be followed with strict discipline.

Yoga was devised by our ancestors thousands of years ago for the benefit of masses to lead a life with a purpose. It was 'Dattatreya' who conceptualised the yoga, 'Sanaka' mastered it and 'Patanjali' laid down the principles of yoga. At that time the main purpose was to explore the Self, serve the society particularly the underprivileged and disabled members of the society, while remaining connected with the higher energies, which were called God. The emphasis was to live this life in harmony with ourselves, our family, community and nature (environment), giving a meaningful purpose to this life.

Yoga is a Sanskrit word which means "to connect". At that time this connection was envisaged to be the connection between the creature and the creator. With education, scientific and technological advancement the definition of yoga has been modified from time to time. In modern world we are dragged by our senses towards luxuries and purpose of life has been changed to earn money and acquire luxuries.

When yoga was invented, that period was dominated by the Jupiter, which is a planet of wisdom, knowledge, good deeds and spirituality.

This was followed by a period dominated by Mars, a planet of strength, wars, might and dictatorship.

During this period lots of wars were fought, masses were suppressed and small countries/kingdoms were created which were ruled by mighty kings.

This was followed by a period dominated by Mercury which is a planet for intellect. During this period evolution advanced further, people became intelligent, the number of intellectuals increased all over the world, scientific discoveries were made, and technological advancement took place.

Since Mercury and Venus are situated near each other and have a relationship of lover and beloved, so luxuries started creeping in. Venus is a planet of richness, luxuries, sex, nakedness and vehicles. Hence we are passing through combined period of Mercury/ Venus which is gradually culminating into the period of Ketu, which is responsible for crimes, deaths, murders, forgery, scams, etc. Ketu also paves the way for spirituality and may lead us to the period of Jupiter once again in not very distant future, where the evolution shall advance further.

Yoga, as mentioned above, means "to connect". To connect:

- The individual soul with eternal soul.
- The human body and mind with the Supreme (God).
- The Microcosm (Human body) with the Macrocosm (Universe).
- The right hemisphere of the brain (right hemisphere of the brain represents female energy which is involved in recognition of patterns, intuition and creative abilities) with the left hemisphere of the brain, which

represents male energy, which is responsible for rationalisation, critical thinking and analytical sense.

- Human Vital Energy with the Cosmic Mother Energy.
- Your lower self (representing senses and illusion) with your higher self (representing the Cosmos or Universe).

  (The higher self has no ego, has no discrimination, it is always one and connected with the Universe).

Yoga is a way of life. It connects the lower self with the higher self to create Universality. The people who practised yoga were called 'yogis'.

In my view, the purpose of human life is:

- To purify energy within us.
- To purify energies around us.

We are a product of our past deeds (Karmas), deeds of our ancestors (Pittri Karmas) inherited by us through our genes and gunas.

Depending upon these deeds, we take birth in a particular family at a particular place under particular circumstances. Our soul is a part of Universal Cosmic Energy (Mother Energy) and our endeavour should be to purify the energy within us and around us to perfection, while remaining connected to our Mother Energy. This can be achieved by following certain principles described in yoga, which are:

- Ethical disciplines.
- Rules of conduct.
- Health of the physical body.

- Correct breathing process.
- Restraining of the senses.
- Meditation.

Ethical Disciplines

To keep yourself pure and for proper integration in society some ethical disciplines are maintain:

(a) Truthfulness.
(b) Non-Violence.
(c) Non-Stealing.
(d) Non-Coveting.

The roots of these evils are *Greed, Desire* and *Attachment*. Rishi Patanjali has described how to overcome these evils by thinking along five principles. Since his original writings are in Sanskrit, some Sanskrit words have been used in the process.

Ahimsa

Ahimsa means non-violence. It is advocated because we are all creation of the one and the same God. Yogis believe that to destroy or kill anything is an insult to its Creator.

Usually humans take to violence to protect their own interests like their own bodies, loved ones, property, dignity, etc. and subsequently violence results in violence. Once we understand that the strength in us is provided by the same source, which has also created our opponent, then there will be no violence. Violence usually arises out of ignorance and fear. A yogi believes that every creature has the same right to live as he has. Ahimsa leads to freedom from fear and freedom from anger and once these are attained, he gets a grip on himself. He starts visualising all other creatures in the self and sees the self in all other creatures. When a yogi dedicates every action to the Lord then he becomes free from fear of losing his body or his belongings. By losing anger the yogi uses the same energy, which ends up in anger, for elevation of the self and spiritual growth.

Satya

Satya means truth. It is said truth is God and the other name of God is truth. The basic inherent nature of a human being is based upon *truth, love* and *bliss.* The truth should be perfect and absolute, *i.e.* truthfulness should be in thought, word and deed. Non-truth puts you out of gear from your inherent nature. Truthfulness should prevail in all spheres of life and not only in speech. A truthful prayer from a pure heart awakens our higher selves.

Asatya

Asatya means non-truth. Desire to possess and enjoy what belongs to others drives a person towards asatya. This includes misuse, mismanagement, breach of trust, misappropriation, etc. A yogi reduces his physical needs to the minimum. Instead of craving for wealth, fame, enjoyment and power he has a craving for adoring the Lord. The Commandment says "thou *shall not steal."*

Brahmacharya

In the true sense, brahmacharya means self-restraint. It was thought that loss of semen (Oja Energy) leads to death and preservation of semen retains life. As long as the semen was preserved yogis had no fear of death. Sankracharya thought that a brahmachari is a person, who has perfected the study of Vedas, knows all the rules of universe and sees divinity in all. It is a wrong notion that a person, who abstains from sex, is a brahmachari. On the other hand, a brahmachari is one who has perfected the knowledge of divine love, happiness and union of soul with the Mother Energy. Yogis have always been recommended to have a married life because it is impossible to experience divine love without experiencing human love. A yogi established in bramacharya develops a store of vital energy and powerful intellect and can fight any type of injustice. Brahmacharya lights the torch of wisdom.

Aparigraha

Parigraha means hoarding and aparigraha means free from hoarding. If stealing is a sin, so is hoarding. To accumulate things, which a person does not need means depriving others of those things who are in need. Hoarding also means accumulating anything without working for it A yogi thinks that hoarding means lack of faith in self to provide for his future. Lack of faith in self is lack of faith in God. A yogi by observing aparigraha thinks that every thing will come to him by the grace of God at the time of need, by doing so he keeps himself away from the misery of the world. A yogi is ever in the belief that God shall fulfill his needs and protect him forever.

Rules of Conduct

These were devised for individual discipline but are universal in their application. Five main rules of conduct are:

1. Purity
2. Contentment

3. Austerity
4. Study of the Self
5. Dedication to God

Purity

Purity means purity of the body as well as purity of the mind. Throwing out the bad impure energy and taking in the pure energy achieves purity of the body. To eliminate the waste products of different parts of the body, certain yoga asanas were devised for those particular parts and these asanas are synchronised with the breathing so as to replace old energy with the new fresh energy. A regulated breathing process is called pranayam. In this process atmospheric air is breathed into the lungs where it saturates the blood with oxygen (energy). This circulates in the whole body and is taken up by all the cells and tissues of the body in the form of energy for their normal functioning. Pranayam being a very important subject shall be described in a separate chapter in this book.

The mind has to be purified from the impurities of hatred, passion, anger, lust, greed, pride, fear, etc. with love, compassion and adoration, which can be cultivated by the study of the self, this is called *internal cleansing*. In this process the mind becomes flexible and it can be trained to think in one direction (single pointed mind). It is easy for a single pointed mind to become master of the senses.

Another way of supplying the energy to the body is through ingestion of food. Here the purity and type of food is important. A detailed chapter on yogic diet has been added to this book. It will suffice to mention here that food should be taken with the intention of providing energy to the body in the name of the God and should not be taken to satisfy the palate.

One should try to live in harmony with Nature. A yogi always thinks his body to be a dwelling place (home) for his soul and tries his best to keep that home clean and healthy.

Besides food, it is important to choose a place for living. The place should be quiet, free from pollution, protected from the bad elements with pleasant surroundings, where food may be easily procurable. That is why yogis used to make their living places along the banks of rivers, lakes or seashores. Such places are very difficult to find in this modern day and age.

Contentment

Contentment has to be cultivated; a discontented mind is always wandering. If your desires and wants are minimal the contentment comes automatically. Contentment leads to bliss and bliss means knowledge of truth and happiness. Contentment brings about tranquility of the mind. It is usually observed that a one pointed mind is usually a contented mind.

Austerity

To achieve a particular goal in life one needs purity of thought, self-discipline and austerity. This involves character building. There is a constant effort to achieve union with the Divine by burning all the desires, which stand in the way of this goal. Austerity allows a person to be humble and non-violent, making him speak the truth, creating a balanced mind, which leads to self-control. This is service without expecting any reward.

Study of the Self

Study of the self means educating the self. This can be gained by either listening to a Guru (teacher) or by meditating on the self.

A person involved in the study of self reads his own book of life while writing it. There is a gradual change in his outlook; he starts adoring the creation, thinks that all creation is divine. All the energies within him, surrounding him and the universal cosmic energy come from one source. One should pursue the study of self throughout one's life because there are always higher goals to be achieved. With the study of the self one needs to study other sacred books and compare his achievements or try to find out the solutions to his problems. This will take away ignorance and bring in knowledge. Once a person attains knowledge of the soul, his faith and beliefs become firmer. The study of the self also makes a yogi aware of the human psychology and working of a normal human mind.

Dedication to God

A yogi always dedicates all his actions to God because he who has faith in God does not despair. He does not want name, fame or power and does not stoop for selfish motives. Excess of energy in the body without proper direction culminates in failure.

A yogi sheds his pride and ego to become one with God, the word 'I' and 'mine' have no meaning for him. There are no desires; the mind is filled with the thoughts of doing everything in the name of God and pleasing him. The name of the Lord shines bright in his mind like the sun taking away all the darkness and sorrows. Once the yogi has learnt the art of dedicating all his actions to the almighty God, Divinity starts reflecting in him.

Health of the Physical Body

Health of the physical body is more important because a non-healthy body cannot function properly. A supple and flexible body is desirable to produce mental equilibrium and a sharp mind. As described earlier, the physical body can be maintained in good shape by performing yoga asanas on a regular basis, which have been described in detail in a separate chapter.

A yogi does not think his physical body is separate from his senses, mind, intellect and soul. By performing yoga asanas regularly, a yogi makes his body a fit vehicle for the soul.

A yogi is never afraid of death. He is fully aware that the body is constantly decaying and death is but a natural process. The soul changes its dwelling place like we change our old and worn-out garments. A yogi understands fully well that this body has been provided to him by the almighty God for his own enjoyment, for serving his near and dear ones and fellowmen, and for serving his Mentor. He never considers this body as the personal property of his soul.

Yoga asanas keep the different parts of the body in a healthy and fit state, which in turn create a complete equilibrium between Body, Mind and Spirit. By doing so he creates the kingdom of God within himself. Body, mind and spirit are interrelated and cannot be separated, while the body is in a perfect state of health. One cannot create a state of equilibrium with his Mother Energy (Universal Cosmic Energy) unless one has a healthy physical body.

Correct Breathing Process

Correct breathing is so much important for the energy system of the body and its maintenance, that a separate chapter has been added to this book called systematic control of the breath (Pranayam). It is the breath which provides maximum energy to the body.

Restraining of the Senses

The physical body derives all its pleasure through the five senses, *i.e.* touch, smell, taste, vision (eyesight) and hearing. A yogi does not let his senses run wild, because anything which is not restrained and not properly guided can go haywire.

By restraining, a yogi directs his sexual energies towards attainment of consciousness. The sense of smell excites the sense of touch, taste as well as vision. A yogi tries to preserve the sense of smell but restrains it from exciting the other senses. A yogi always tries to use his sense of hearing for hearing good things about others, for hearing praises of the Lord and for enjoying nature. A yogi uses his sense of vision to appreciate the creation of nature and to convey messages through his visual sense. A yogi uses his sense of taste for keeping the body healthy and in a fit state, by restraining his sense to eat to live and not live to eat.

Meditation

This is one of the most important processes for a yogi. A separate chapter on Yoga Energy System which also includes meditation, its effects on the body and mind has been added to this book. Readers who wish to start meditation from the beginning are referred to the author's book, *Vital Energy*.

Evolution and Yoga

1

EVOLUTION AND YOGA

Evolution is defined in Oxford Dictionary as a gradual change in characteristics of a population over successive generations. It may be applied to an individual or an individual organ, like brain. Individual evolution takes place by the theory of one soul and many bodies in successive births in the process of Reincarnation.

According to one of the most accepted theories, the origin of the human species took place in *East African Savannah,* where the ancestors of modern man used to live.

The theory that humans descended from apes is widely accepted whereas apes themselves evolved from more primitive mammals. Humans not only look like apes, they think like apes. Over millions of years, some of the emotions and reactions we exhibit still have the impressions of Stone Age. It seems that these characters are imprinted in our make-up. We still exhibit those characters which our ancestors had millions of years ago, like instincts of survival, aggression, competition and Procraetion. We still grope in the dark when we think about ourselves. Who are we? Why are we here? What hidden treasures we possess?

Before I proceed further, I would like to explain a few terms, which will be frequently used in the following pages.

Savannah: Open grassland, usually with scattered bushes or trees, characteristic of tropical Africa and some parts of Australia.

Australopithecus: Any of the various extinct ape-like primates whose remains have been found in southern and eastern Africa, some of them upto 4.5 million years old.

Homohabilis: Species of primates of Genus Homo, including Man.

Homo erectus: Homo genus standing on hind legs.

Homo: Same or similar.

Homogeneous: Composed of similar or identical parts or elements. It also means similarity in structure because of common ancestory. All primates belong to Genus Homogeneous, including Man.

Primates: Placental mammals, having flexible hands, good eyesight and highly developed brain. Primates include lemurs, apes and man.

Homo sapiens: Modern man including primitive man, such as Cro-Magnon man, which is an extinct species.

Trait: A characteristic feature distinguishing a particular person or thing.

Instinct: Inborn intuitive power?

Intuition: Knowledge or perception not gained by reasoning. It is based on knowledge gained in our previous lives, cosmic connections, and also during the present life.

Altruism: Selfless service or service with no personal motive?

We began life on the Savannah as Australopithecus, with the brain size of Chimpanzee (300 gms) over 4.5 million years ago, over the next 3 million years this brain tripled in size. As we grew the way we are now, the number of brain cells increased. At present our brain has around one hundred billion nerve cells.

Mind which is created by brain is increasingly getting complex and sophisticated. We are evolving more curiosity for learning, emotions and rationality, but it does not mean that we have completely lost our animal instinct.

When we reached Stone Age, we learnt to make tools, discovered fire and its uses and started to explore. We started talking and communicating, we also started living in groups, although we had learned this as animals, that to protect ourselves it was essential to live in a group to ward off dangers, but those groups now became larger. We started pooling information about the environment, water, food and fuel. Larger groups became feasible knitted by emotional threads and the will to cooperate, eventually it led us to trace our roots, build civilisations and invent cultural life.

Increasing emotions led us towards material wealth, but lots of emotional needs were still not fulfilled.

We were forced, as a species, to inherit genetic traits from the life we had led for over 4.5 million years of "Savannah psychology". These traits preceded our Hominids stage .The mind we are born with is different from the mind developed by learning, culture, socialisation.

Instinct is that part of behaviour of mind, with which we are born, but the environment may affect the way the instincts are expressed. Desire, reasoning and behaviour are inherited. Specifically human instincts were ingrained in us during our time on the Savannah.

Instincts are embedded in us in the form of genetic coding, in the strands of DNA in our genes. Recently DNA technology has advanced so much, it is being used in so many spheres of life. Within the DNA code lies the recipe for the development of the human body.

This code is identical in most human beings. There is, however, minute variation which makes us different from others, and explains the variation in human physiology, hormonal balance, tendency to get various diseases and coloration of the skin and iris (eyes).

Development of the human brain is determined largely by this genetic code, but working of different brains is still a mystery.

Man has been an animal since he walked first, more than 4 million years ago. For 2 million years he was a tribal warrior/hunter. Social drives developed long before we developed intellectually. It is this *intellect* which separates us from animals. Intellect is also developed in certain animals. Intellect developed as the control over the instincts increased.

Humans are designed to modify their behaviour according to circumstances; this is called *self-discipline* which differentiates humans from lower animals. More self-discipline makes humans refined and less discipline takes them towards lower animals who are driven by their instincts. Genetically there is only 2 per cent difference between humans and apes.

Facial features changed to the modern appearance about 100,000 years ago. Early humans had all the instincts of animals. They lived in small groups, which meant that they could ward off dangers together with strength. They lived in caves and were carnivorous, either they killed their own prey or they acted as scavengers to the animals killed by big cats or other stronger animals. Their brain had increased in size to 600-800 grams. They knew how to mate and produce offsprings/children. Males were much bigger than females. Females needed protection and food which was provided by males. There were no marriages. The children belonged to the tribe. There were fights among the tribes for territory and mating with females, killings took place and there was bloodshed.

Our ancestors were driven to eat better quality proteins and fat derived from meat. Animals like cows and rabbits that were herbivorous and ate greens and vegetables required a longer gut to digest them. Our ancestors learned to cook to make food palatable; cooking also made meat and vegetables easily digestible, hence they needed shorter gut. Gut in humans became shorter but brain became bigger. Along with the increase in size of the brain the head size also increased. From infancy to adulthood the brain size increases fourfold. With the increase in head size, there took place changes in the female pelvis, so as to allow the passage of fetal head from the birth canal at the time of delivery. Labour is a painful process in females due to the size of the human fetal head. The extraordinary growth of brain defined our evolutionary path which is a 5 million years long story.

A larger brain does not mean better intelligence, but it can perform more sophisticated functions. A larger brain had advantages for early humans. It is known that people with larger brain were able to survive and reproduce. A larger brain developed better instincts and skills which were used for hunting.

In Stone Age, humans developed weapons from stones to kill their prey from a distance, an example of such a weapon is Frisbee. They also developed weapons to skin the animals of prey. Later an important tool was added, *i.e.* hand axe which had multiple uses.

Still later analytical skills were developed like reasoning and logic. These skills were developed gradually, because the bigger brain had more surface area, more connections, and more cells called neurons which formed more connections.

Out of all the human instincts, the sex instinct is the most important. We are obsessed with sex. It is embedded in human nature to pass on the genes to the next generation.

Life in Savannah was always on sword's edge, there was fear of being attacked by animals, fear of war between different tribes, fear of disease and sickness. In the 19th century "Charles Darwin" of England put forward his theory of "Natural Selection", the "Survival of the fittest". After birth all species struggle to survive, but only the fittest survive, the rest are perished or eaten by bigger animals. In 1852, "Herbert Spencer", a colleague of Darwin, said that human society was also subject to the process of natural selection like animals.

As Time passed by, humans became refined, they formed society and recognised sex as a necessity and they began looking for a mate. Women who were young, fertile and healthy had better chances of bearing a number of children. Men in all cultures, therefore, found younger women more sexually attractive. Men wanted attractive women, whereas women did not bother for the looks, they looked for security, stability and long lasting relationship. Males were big and tall, but females were small and short. Genetically it is embedded in male human genes to prefer symmetrical faces. Males wanted young women with proportionate bodies as mates to propagate their genes to the next generation.

Humans developed intelligence and used it for exploring. They started exploring the earth for better food, better living conditions, better mates, and better climate, as the climate at Savannah was very hot. They started travelling far and wide and settled at those places where they found the conditions congenial and suitable. Most of the settlements were near a water source, as water was essential for life.

A tribe called *Aryans* came and settled along a river called 'Sindu' which was located in an area, now known as South East Asia. I shall describe this tribe in greater details in the subsequent pages.

Exchange of information, gossip, and its means go back to 1.5 million years. Social intelligence played a role in increasing the brain size and developed intuitive sense. Brains are so expensive to build and maintain.

'Lambroso' was a well known criminologist who was born in Verona and his work was published in 1876. He believed that ancient humans were much more violent and criminal minded than modern men. Modern criminals not only shared their ancestors' criminal tendencies, but also their physical appearance. The criminal man was essentially an evolutionary degenerate.

Humans are essentially self-centered. They however cooperate with the society to gain more food, sex, status for themselves. They also want/demand protection from enemies and environmental hardships. But there are proofs that homo sapiens also cared for the weak and vulnerable.

Bonobos who are closely related to chimpanzees and are thought to be man's closest living relatives have been observed to care for the weak and vulnerable.

"Franz de Wall" and "Jessica Flack" are convinced that human morality has deep roots in our primate past. It is beyond doubt that we are creatures of intellect. It is also clear that we are born with powerful inclinations and emotions that bias our thinking and behaviour

About 20000-30000 years ago the elders and intellectuals of the tribes decided to reform their way of living and way of thinking, prior to that humans thought that they were supreme amongst the living creatures. But when they could not understand some phenomenon of the nature, they were compelled to alter their thinking. They thought that there was a Creator who was Supreme who created this Universe including mountains, rivers, jungle/forests, other planets, etc and they gave him the name of God. Intellectuals meditated to find answers to some of many questions from God, the Creator, the Sustainer, the Destroyer, because Death was inevitable. Nobody great or small was saved from the clutches of Death.

Tribes became larger. The communities were taught to live in harmony with each other. Marriage was introduced, so as to increase loyalty and sharing of emotions and to produce pure progeny *i.e.* high quality offspring.

Evolution can not be brought about by only mutation of genes, external factors also influence it. These external factors include past karmas(deeds), bringing up, family, status of the family / individual in the society, socialisation and environment in which we live, etc. These external factors constitute 'Prakriti' whereas our genetic factors along with our past karmas make up 'Gunas'!

Hindu mythology believes that the entire cosmos is evolved from Prakriti and Prakriti is made of three qualities (Gunas), which correspond with Matter, Energy and Consciousness, which guide our lives. All of us are born with all three Gunas, but a particular Guna dominates depending upon the accumulated karmas of our past births, karmas of our ancestors embedded in our genes and even karmas of our community (racial characters). Our whole existence is based on these Gunas called Sattva, Rajas and Tamas.

Sattva is truth, essence or God like. It represents mind or consciousness. A pure mind leads to self-realisation. A pure mind is Sattva and Sattva is divine nature. A divine mind explores inwards and tries to unify heart and brain. Sattva is a spiritual quality which represents love, peace, intelligence and harmony, which makes the soul rise upwards towards realisation and liberation. Upwards represents the logic which is the function of the brain.

Sattva is nectar, which in the body is represented by secretions of pineal gland, pituitary gland and hypothalamus, which are all situated in the brain.

Sattvic people eat very little, just to survive. They prefer nourishing, simple, natural foods which are low in calories like fresh milk, fresh vegetables, fruits, nuts and wheat. They perform actions without being attached to their results; their actions are performed keeping all the community in mind. They meditate for the betterment of the community. Their lives are dedicated to the community/society.

Rajas represent a turbulent mind, which looks outwards to seek fulfillment of desires. Rajasic mind is agitated by anger, manipulativeness and egoistic attitude. Rajasic mind seeks power through fair means or foul. Rajas represent energy at subtle plain. Rajas' qualities are action, turbulance, passion, aggression, competition, pain and strife. They become mad for worldly possessions and gains. These qualities keep the soul in the middle world which means attachments, acquisitions and achievements. Rajasic people are impatient to achieve the desired results. They love the food which tickles their taste buds, is high in calories and gives a lot of energy like meat, milk products, wheat, cooked vegetables, etc.

Tamas is inertia, dullness, ignorance. A tamas mind is an ignorant mind which lacks activity and sensitivity and is dominated by external subconscious forces leading to primitive animal nature including lack of personal hygiene.

Tamas represents matter at physical plane which is darkness, obstruction and lethargy; it is animal quality that keeps the soul in lower worlds. It creates decay and destruction harmful to others. Tamas people eat anything which comes in their way like half cooked, stale, leftover food, which are more acidic and non-nourishing.

Sattva and tamas are two sides of the same coin. If sattva is nectar then tamas is poison, represented by metabolic waste of the body. When you remove bad qualities from the poison, it becomes nectar, if bad qualities are added to the nectar it becomes poison.

Rajas and tamas go hand in hand. When rajas gets in excess, it depletes energy through over activity and makes one tamasic *i.e.* lethargic and dull. Rajas creates energy, vitality and emotions, whereas tamas creates energy that allows fixed ideas to take shape. Rajas is a bridge between sattva and tamas, it can change sattva into tamas and vice versa. Because rajasic energy produces illusion, if rajas is controlled anything'can be achieved. Rajas act with passion guided by desire, tamas act without thinking, whereas Sattvas are guided by intuition.

Humans from Savannah migrated to different parts of the planet Earth. As mentioned earlier, the community called "Aryans", who came and settled along the banks of river 'Sindhu', came to be known as Hindus eventually. They developed their own means of survival, own means of communication and the language they developed came to be known as Sanskrit. They also developed their means of transportation, warfare, sophistication and spirituality for communication with their higher self or universal cosmic energy called God. The description you will read in subsequent pages relates to the development of this community only.

Humans have attempted to create legal systems since the beginning of recorded history. According to records Humurali established some legal system and moral codes about 2000 B.C. There were 282 law codes and most of them were meant to organise the society.

Law protected the integrity of the family unit. Virtually every single system of ethics invented, tried to find a way to provide good reason to banish selfishness and work in the interest of other members of the community.

'Ehrlich', a Swedish scientist, says that capacity to construct a moral system is a product of human evolution. We can envisage the consequences of our actions, think of alternatives and imagine the feelings of others. All these are valuable qualities and with our *Free Will* are preconditioned for creating a moral system, which will be the outcome of human culture.

With the increase in the brain size, the instincts of 'Hindus' changed, their imagination increased. Their imagination and intuitive powers developed with meditation to communicate with the cosmos/nature. They thought of creating a civilised and disciplined society. It was essential to guide the public at large, for that intellectuals of the society devised a way of spending life, which came to be known as *Yog*. This system had everything including the moral code, physical fitness, mental/psychological fitness, advice regarding diet/food, sexual activity, etc. In short yoga explained everything: How to lead a pure and honest life, remaining connected with your higher self *i.e.*univesal cosmic energy/mother energy (God), by following the laws of the nature.

Every thing was devised keeping the then society and prakriti in mind. With the changing scenario in the world, people moulded yoga according to their needs and wishes, but time has proved that principles laid at that time hold well to this day, because they are based on realities of life and Universal Laws, which will hold good for millions of years to come.

They divided the community/society into different categories, depending upon their stage of evolution, intellect, physique, nature and Gunas. These categories were called "VERNAS". Better evolved people with superior intellect, who could comprehend the knowledge of their higher self/God, were called 'Brahmanas'. Brahamna means a person who has knowledge of the Supreme and can anticipate the events to come. Highly intellectual and intuitive persons were called 'Rishis'.They were assigned the duty to guide the society, teach the rules of Dharma and to discipline it. Their thinking, actions were simple but nurturing. They showed compassion and had a 'Sattvic' disposition. They had well-developed left brain and critically analysed everything. They were appointed as advisers to the rulers/kings.

People with robust physique, who had aggressive characters, who ate high calorie animal food, who were less compassionate, who had developed rapid thinking (usually they acted before thinking of the consequences), in short who believed in Do or Die and had a 'Rajasic' disposition, were assigned the duty to protect the society and Dharma. They were hard-core people, mainly fighters and were taught the fighting skills by Gurus (MASTER) who were Brahmanas.They made good orators, rulers, fighters, and were skilled in warfare. They were called 'Kashatrias'. Although they were predominantly left brain users, there was less logic and more action in their karmas. The uppermost instinct in their mind was to win, be it war, women or wealth. They protected the Dharma rules by hook or by crook.

People who fitted in between Brahmans and Kashatrias,who had comparatively less evolved brains but moderate physique, reasonable thinking power and who had sharp analytical left brain, were assigned the duty to maintain the society. They were providers of the society. They had sattva and rajas, gunas equally balanced. They were tradesmen, who had the responsibility to feed and maintain the society in good as well as bad times *i.e.* during wars and natural calamities. They were called 'Vaishyas'.

People at lower level of evolution, with weak physique who were unable to perform brainy jobs, who had less developed thinking process and were unable to take initiatives, were called 'Sudras'. They were assigned menial tasks and were given the privilege to serve the other three classes of the society, so that they could devote more time to their allotted tasks and excel in them. Sudras were manual labourers, poor thinkers and lethargic by nature. Their basic needs were survival and security which was provided by the rest of the society.

Another view is that this part of the world which is called Indian subcontinent now has always been very fertile, rich in natural resources and rich in culture too; hence it has been a target for invasion by foreigners from time immemorial.

According to Western historians this land was invaded by Aryans 4000-5000 years B.C. ago who came from across the Himalayas and fought the 'Dravidians' (who had invaded the area before them)and the original inhabitants. To maintain purity of race, Aryans created their own social order and divided the community which was the beginning of Caste system in India.

Aryans were Indo-Europeans or 'Caucasians' were the creators of great Hindu civilisation.

Rig Veda tells the story of long struggle between Aryans and aboriginal people of Indian subcontinent.

Aryans first invaded Northern India and since they were from European region, they were white, but they enslaved the local aboriginal inhabitants who were black and called them 'Shudras' and gradually the order developed with whites on the top, mixed race in the middle and blacks on the bottom to serve the others.

For generations black Indians have served their white bosses. Colour orientated, racially based Caste system became the foundation of the religion which came to be known as 'Hinduism'.

According to Indian historians, *Aryans* were original inhabitants of Northern India and *Dravidians* were inhabitants of the South, both had the same culture and coexisted. Language of both *Aryans* and *Dravidians* was sanskrit and as they evolved the society evolved. In olden days the Hindu land was called *Arya Vrat,* which was changed to *Bharat Varash* during the regimen of King Bharta. Muslims in seventh century gave the name *Hindustan,* which means a place where Hindus live. English rulers in eighteenth century A.D. called it *India,* after the Indus Valley, where Hindus were settled predominantly.

Perhaps in other parts of the world, such refinements in the society were taking place but because of inadequate means of transportation and lack of communication, people living in various parts of the world were not aware of the happenings in the other communities. People were scattered in communities which were enlarging all over the earth and were trying to demarcate their boundaries and had devised their own rules of living depending upon the natural resources available in their areas/regions.

The Hindu community decided to integrate itself by framing certain rules. Hindus came up with the theory of "Common Source", *i.e.* all humans are from a common source that is universal cosmic energy, which they called 'God'. All of them owed something to each other, so they should work for mutual interests. They wanted to convert the self-centered Man to the society-centered creature. The class system was created keeping this in mind, so that everybody worked, dedicating all actions to God, for mutual interest of the society.

Yog or Yoga may be defined as a way of life, in which every individual act was performed for the benefit of all members of the society, keeping in mind our common source of existence. The act was performed while remaining connected with the mother energy and in her name.

PHYSICAL REJUVENATION

2

Physical Rejuvenation

Since the physical body represents *matter,* it is the dwelling place of the soul representing *energy*. It is the energy, which gives life to the physical body. Like any other dwelling place it is our duty to keep the dwelling place of the soul in clean and healthy environment/ condition. *Mind* also lives in the body. Thought process originates in the mind. Thinking process is very important for the purity of the soul. To keep the soul (energy) pure it is essential to have a stable and relaxed mind and for this a healthy body is essential. In yoga, some definitive ways have been described to achieve this, which are:

(a) *Regular bathing,* it is essential to keep the undesirable elements like dirt, bacteria, and waste products thrown out on the surface of the body by the process of sweating, to be washed away from the external surface of the body. Regular bathing not only cleans the body surface, but it also opens up the pores in the skin, making them breathe in an orderly manner, providing energy to the body.

(b) *Nourishment,* it is necessary to provide the body with the constant nourishments so as to produce the required energy necessary for the functioning of the body.

(i) It can be achieved by taking food at appropriate intervals.

(ii) It is also achieved by proper breathing in which we draw the energy from the atmosphere.

(iii) By bathing the body in the sun because the best source of energy for the human body comes from the sun, which has so many energising factors including heat. To understand fully the energy system of the body the reader is referred to the author's book, *Vital Energy*.

(c) *Yoga Asanas* (different postural exercises), to keep different parts and systems of the body in a healthy and fit state so that they can perform their normal functions in a regulated manner, Yoga recommends certain exercises (asanas) to be performed on a regular basis. A separate chapter describing some of the procedures in detail has been included in this book.

(d) *Pranayam* (breathing exercises), these are recommended for regulating and controlling the energy being supplied and circulating in the body. A separate chapter describing certain procedures in detail has been included in this book.

Asanas versus exercises

The main difference between an exercise and an asana is that an exercise is done haphazardly whereas an asana is performed with proper sequence and the mind responds to every sequence. In other words, in a yoga asana, mind cannot be separated from the act whereas in an ordinary exercise mind is far off from the act. In an asana, stretching of a group of muscles is always followed by relaxation of those muscles, whereas in an ordinary exercise it may not happen.

Performance of yoga asanas are based on the following set principles, which are:

(1) Mind should go with each and every act of Asana. It is desirable to relax the mind to the extent of meditation point.

(2) When an asana is performed, in which a group of muscles is contracted (tensed), it should always be followed by relaxation of those muscles.

(3) Giving rest to the body or part of the body is an essential element between the performances of two different yoga asanas. The time spent on performing an asana should preferably be the same as the time spent on resting the body after the asana.

(4) Evacuation of the bowels regularly, once or twice a day, is very important because according to yoga, body functions go into disarray if the waste products are not expelled from the body.

(5) Proper breathing techniques are followed to synchronise with each act of asana. When a muscle or a group of muscles are performing (contracted), it is synchronised with inhalation (breathing the air in) because muscles / tissues need more energy when they are performing, whereas relaxation of a muscle or a group of muscles is synchronized with exhalation (breathing the air out).

(6) Asanas are performed to keep the particular part of the body mobile and flexible.

(7) In yoga asanas, maximum importance is given to the mobility of the spine (backbone) for two reasons:

   (a) All the nerves, which supply energy to different parts of the body, come out of the

spinal cord which runs in the centre of the spine. If the spine or the bones forming the spine (backbone), becomes stiff it is likely to put pressure on those nerve roots, disrupting the functions of those parts to which those nerves supply energy.

(b) Maximum flow of the energy in the bioplasmic body is along the spine because all the major chakras (man holes of energy) are situated along the spine. A diseased or a stiff spine may lead to interruption in the flow of the energy, disrupting the entire energy system of the body.

To keep the body fit should be our prime job because a diseased body leads to a worried mind and a worried mind is not capable of thinking efficiently. The inclination of a worried mind is always towards negativity. Negative thoughts agitate the nerves which in turn lead to tense muscles. A body which becomes repeatedly tense succumbs to disease.

I wish to assure the readers that nobody has died of physical exhaustion (due to physical overwork), but I have come across people dying of mental exhaustion, because mental exhaustion leads to physical exhaustion whereas vice versa is not true.

Most of the religions teach us methods to purify the body. A purified body is a fit body. Religions also tell us that this body does not belong to us; it is given to us by God and is returned to God when we die. We act as keepers of this body during our lifetime and it becomes our duty to keep this body healthy and fit as far as we can. This may be achieved by keeping ourselves as close to Mother Nature as possible.

Industrialisation has not only taken us away from Mother Nature but has led to the pollution of the air we breathe, the food we eat, and has also polluted our minds. We have forgotten the aim for which we are born. We have made money as our goal in life and are prepared to do anything to achieve that, to the extent that we are even prepared to sell Mother Nature for the sake of money. We do not realise that money is an essential evil and is the root cause of all the problems in the world. It can only satisfy the desires produced by the Prakriti (external nature) but cannot satisfy the hunger of our inner nature (true nature).

For keeping the body fit it is essential to have a calm mind, because a calm mind leads to a calm body. In this chapter I am going to describe the ways and means for keeping the body fit.

Yoga Asanas

Yogis have described certain postures called yoga asanas to activate different groups of muscles, hence keeping different parts of the body in a fit and energized state. I do not have any intention to write a treatise on yoga asanas, but I intend to describe a few asanas in detail so that any person who wishes to perform them on a regular basis can keep his body in a fit state.

Definition

Yog asanas are various exercises which are performed to get rid of the waste products of different parts of the body in the form of bad energy and to replenish those parts with fresh energy. The asanas are also a means of gaining steadiness of position and success in contemplation, without distracting the mind.

The slightest discomfort/pain during an asana will draw the mind away and it will only return to a peaceful state when the cause of the pain has ceased.

Yoga asanas versus physical exercises

The main differences between yoga asnas and ordinary physical exercises are:

(1) Yoga asanas are performed in a certain sequence and rhythm whereas physical exercises are non-sequential and non-rhythmic. In a yoga asana, the mind follows the rhythm but in a physical exercise it is independent of the act.

(2) During exercises the body parts become stiff due to uneven pressure, hence the mind starts wandering, whereas yoga asanas produce elasticity in the body keeping the mind aligned with the act. If the mind is not with the act the effect of a yoga asana is reduced.

(3) During exercises the breathing process remains independent of the act and the performer becomes breathless. The sequences of yoga asanas are always synchronised with the breathing.

(4) During exercises the ductless glands of the body are unevenly influenced. Yoga asanas influence the glands evenly and in a regulated manner, so that they secrete the juices in an orderly manner and pour them in the general circulation.

(5) In most of the physical exercises it is the skeletal muscles, which are exercised whereas in yoga asanas even the internal organs are exercised.

(6) Physical exercises influence the physical body, whereas yoga asanas influence the physical body as well as the energy (bioplasmic) body.

(7) Physical exercises leave a person exhausted. Yoga asanas relieve fatigue and leave the body energised and light.

(8) A lot of importance has been given to seminal fluid in yoga. Physical exercises help in the release of the seminal fluid which is pushed downwards and outwards. Yoga asanas help in pushing the seminal fluid upwards converting the sexual energy into Ojas (spiritual energy).

(9) At the end of physical exercises one feels tired, exhausted, lethargic and sleepy whereas after performing yoga asanas one feels energised, alive and kicking, fresh and active.

(10) Physical exercises make the muscles tense and joints stiff, yoga asanas relax the muscles and make the joints pliable and supple.

Do's & Don'ts for performing yoga asanas

Do's

(1) Always prepare your mind before starting a yoga asana. Preparation of the mind means bringing the mind into the act and not allowing it to wander away.

(2) Either taking in a deep breath or breathing out precedes every act in a yoga asana. Synchronising every act of asana with breathing is an important part of yoga asanas; because it is through the process of breathing that we throw out the bad energy and take

in the good (fresh) energy. It is always advisable to breathe through the nose, as breathing through the mouth can make your mouth and tongue dry making the act uncomfortable.

(3) Regularity in performance of the asanas is not only important but also essential, because once a joint/ a group of muscles is trained to relax it is likely to go back to its original position if that training is not followed at regular intervals. It is advocated that yoga asanas should be performed every day. According to the author's experience one day off in a week does a lot of good. to the body to regain fresh energy.

(4) While performing yoga asanas it is preferable that every asana is followed by a resting asana. During the act of the an asana part gets rid of the waste products/ bad energy, while during the resting asana it regains fresh energy.

(5) Yoga asanas should always be performed with your eyes closed, because by doing so you partially cut the mind from outside distractions and allow it to follow the act of the asana.

(6) Always try to perform yoga asanas after emptying your bladder and evacuating your bowels, by doing so you will be saved of the interruptions of the calls of the nature.

Don'ts

(1) Never perform asanas in a hurry, as the purpose of the asanas is not served and

chances of injury to that particular part of the body are increased.

(2) While performing a yoga asana never exceed the tolerance of the body; again you can harm that particular part.

(3) It is advised not to perform any yoga asana with a full stomach, so asanas are not performed after meals. It is preferable to have an interval of 4 hours for performing asanas after a meal. There is only one exception and that is Vajar Asana, which is performed 20 minutes to half an hour after taking meals, because this asana is particularly helpful in process of digestion of the food.

(4) Always avoid asanas during early pregnancy and in the last two months of pregnancy as well as two weeks after confinement. By early pregnancy I mean the first eight weeks after conception, because chances of miscarriage are increased. It is quite safe to perform yoga asanas from the ninth week to 32 weeks of pregnancy. There are special asanas which are performed to strengthen the pelvic muscles.

(5) Special precautions are advised for people suffering from heart trouble, high blood pressure and chronic diseases of the lungs. These precautions will be mentioned with individual asanas.

(6) In olden days, yoga asanas were not recommended to be performed by women who were menstruating, but with modern modified techniques this is now safe.

Preparation for performing yoga asanas

- Yoga asanas should always be performed with pure body and calm mind.
- Asanas are best performed at a quiet open place, preferably surrounded by plants and trees with plenty of fresh air as fresh air contains a higher percentage of oxygen.
- Asanas should be performed preferably at dawn, because the plants and trees start releasing oxygen as soon as light falls on them. Oxygen is a vital component of the energy system of the human body.
- Asanas may also be performed around sunset.
- Asanas may be performed while sitting, standing or lying. One should select a level piece of ground on which one can spread a durrie or a mat, which should be comfortable while sitting or lying.
- One should sit upright preferably in the lotus position with eyes closed and try to concentrate, repeating inside, "I am going to perform this act to remain healthy", and this should be repeated till you reach the meditation point.
- By closing the eyes the mind is taken away from external distractions and is made to look/ concentrate on the act being performed.
- If mind and body are completely relaxed it is nice to start the whole episode with a prayer to the Almighty.
- Asanas for relaxing different parts of the body will be described in the subsequent chapters.

- Concentration on breathing is a necessary requirement for performance of yoga asanas.

Daily plan for rejuvenation of the body

I plan to give a regimen by which one can keep different parts of the body healthy and fit. The whole process entails sparing one hour in the morning. Those individuals who do not have easy excess to a park or an open space can perform this regimen in their drawing rooms / homes. The regimen is as follows:

Step 1: Sit in an upright position keeping the back straight with folded legs or preferably sit in the lotus position (this position shall be described in detail in subsequent paragraphs), with eyes closed , concentrate your mind on your breath. Once your breath becomes rhythmic or attains a particular rhythm you go into a phase of concentration.

Step 2: Once the rhythm is attained in breathing you should get ready to say a prayer. Prayer may be said silently by opening your heart or may be uttered loudly. You should not be selfish to pray for yourself or for your family; rather you should pray for the whole world. Prayer makes a person humble, creates boundaries for ego, makes a person compassionate and calms the mind.

Step 3: After having said the prayer you should go back to the stage of concentration and try to follow your breath inside your body for 2 to 3 minutes. These three steps should be finished in 5 to 6 minutes.

This is followed by performance of yoga asanas. I suggest that one should perform one asana while standing, one asana while sitting, one asana while kneeling, and one or two asanas while lying on your tummy, one asana while lying on your back and one asana which affects almost all the parts of the body. In between these asanas one has to perform the resting asana which follows each and every asana.

Some of the important asanas are described below:

Lotus Position (Padam Asana)

This is performed in a sitting position. You sit upright with back and neck straight and folded legs; eyes closed and keeping the hand either in the lap or holding the knees (see the photograph). This asana helps in maintaining the posture of the spine correctly. It also helps free flow of breath through the nose to the lungs. This asana energises the Muladhara Chakra (a brief description of this chakra is given in the chapter on Energy), which in turn binds us with Mother Earth, gives us confidence and helps in the growth of the body. This asana helps in the mobility of hip, knee and ankle joints. Yogis commonly adopt the lotus position for meditation, dhyana and Samadhi.

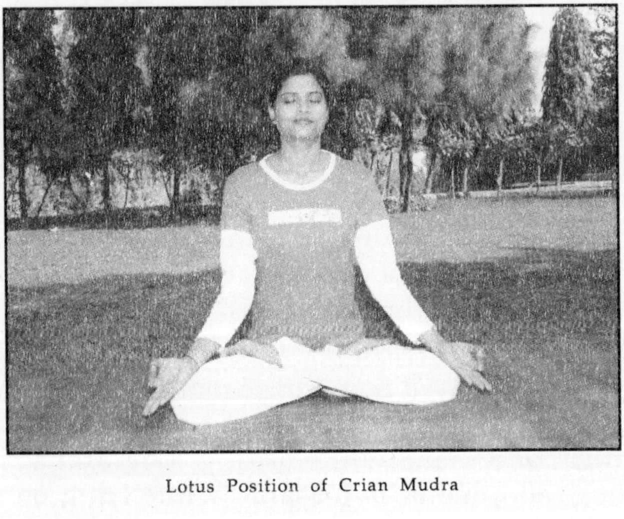

Lotus Position of Crian Mudra

Effects

(1) It helps in keeping the spine in the erect position.

(2) It helps in flexibility of hip, knee and ankle joints.

(3) It stimulates and energises the Muladhara Chakra, where Kundalini Shakti lies in its resting form.

(4) It helps in the free flow of the air utilised during the process of normal breathing.

(5) It also stimulates Manipura Chakra to an extent and helps in the process of digestion.

(6) It helps the energy to ascend upwards, which ultimately helps in relaxation of the nerves and the meditative process.

Caution

People with the following condition should not attempt to sit in the lotus position:

(1) Sick and debilitated people.

(2) Persons suffering from arthritis of the hips, knees or ankles.

(3) Very fat people with large protuberant tummies.

(4) People with abnormalities of the spine (backbone).

Sukh Asana

This is a sitting asana which may be used during meditation, as it allows a person to sit comfortably for a long period.

This may be performed by sitting straight on the bottom keeping the spine and neck in one straight line, the feet are comfortably placed below the opposite knee (as shown in the photograph) and keep the hands in any mudra. The eyes are kept closed and the mind is made steady by pointing it in a single direction. The breath is regulated as in yogic breathing.

Effects

(1) By keeping the mind on the Agya Chakra, you may open your third eye and visualize things.

(2) This asana teaches us to sit in a properly relaxed manner for a long period.

(3) It regulates the process of breathing.

(4) A sustained practice of this asana calms the mind and improves its concentration.

Caution

The same caution which applies to the lotus position.

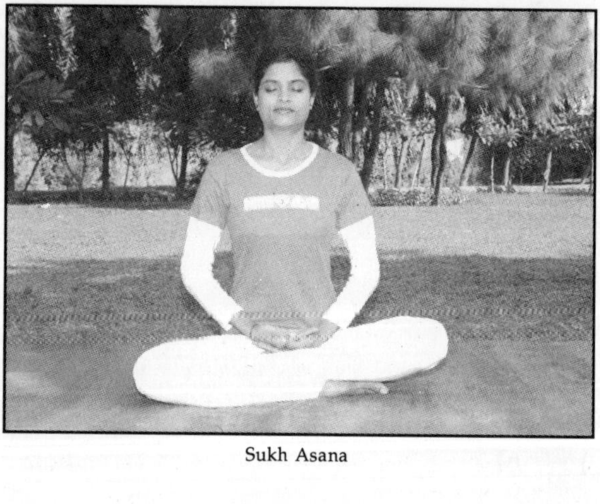

Sukh Asana

Siddh Asana

This is considered to be best posture for meditation. This is performed in a sitting position with bent knees, keeping the left heel between the anus and the genitalia and placing the right heel at the root of the genitalia. In this position, one ankle joint crosses over the other ankle joint and the toes of one foot are placed between the knee fold of the other leg and vice versa. The hands are kept in Gyan mudra whereas the back and the neck are kept straight and eyes are lightly closed.

Effects

(1) Since the Prana moves with the mind in the same direction, this asana being the best meditative pose allows the prana to move upwards which makes the semen also move upwards, hence preserving celibacy.

(2) This asana makes you control your prana and seminal energy, which indirectly influences the senses and makes them look inwards for the pleasure rather than to look outwards.

(3) It is said to be a very good asana for controlling night emissions and unwanted sexual desires.

Caution

The same which applies to the lotus position.

Vajar Asana

This asana is performed while sitting on folded knees; both the knees are completely flexed and are joined together in front whereas both the heels are kept apart slanting to the sides, right foot slightly over riding the left foot. The bottom fits in within both the heels. The

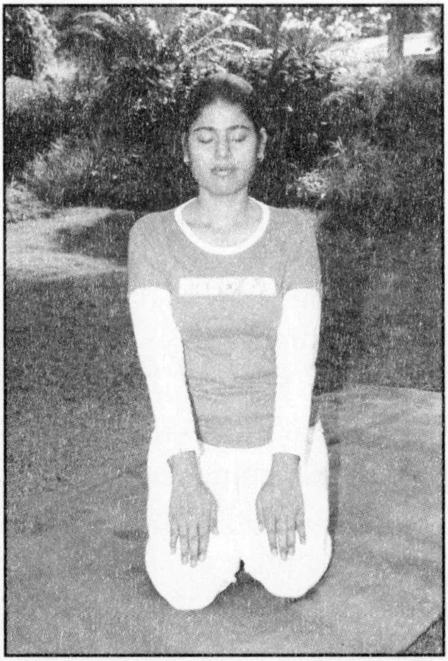

Vajar Asana (Front)

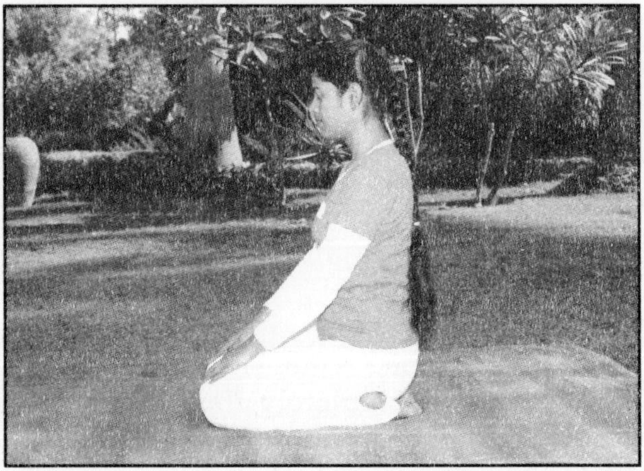

Vajar Asana (Side View)

neck and back are kept straight in upright position, the arms are stretched and hands are kept on the knees, of course the eyes remain shut (see the photograph).

Effects

This asana energises the Manipura Chakra (refer to the chapter on Chakras), which in turn helps in the digestion of the food. This is the only asna, which can be performed after eating food. It is suggested that 15 to 20 minutes after finishing your food you should empty your bladder and sit in Vajar Asana for about 20 minutes, it hastens the process of digestion. This asana also helps in keeping the hip, knee, and ankle joints flexible. Muslims, for saying their prayers, adopt this position.

Caution

Vajar Asana should not be attempted by persons suffering from:

1. Arthritis of the hip, knees or ankle.
2. Arthritis or deformity of the entire spine, particularly the lumbar spine.

Yoga Mudra

This is also performed in a sitting position. Sit in the lotus position, with eyes closed and neck and back straight. Once you are fully grounded try to bring both your heels as near to each other or as near to your tummy as possible. Take both the arms to your back, make a fist of the left hand and hold the left wrist with you right hand, pull both the hands backwards and downwards so as to stretch the spine a bit more. Take a long and a deep breath and fill both the lungs with the air. Gradually bend forward, breathing out, keeping both the arms stretched backwards and downwards, exhaling all the air. Try to touch your forehead with the ground in front of you (see the photographs of different postures). Feel the pressure of both the heels on your liver, stomach, spleen and colon. The asana may be repeated by twisting the spine to right/left and touching your nose to the right/left knee.

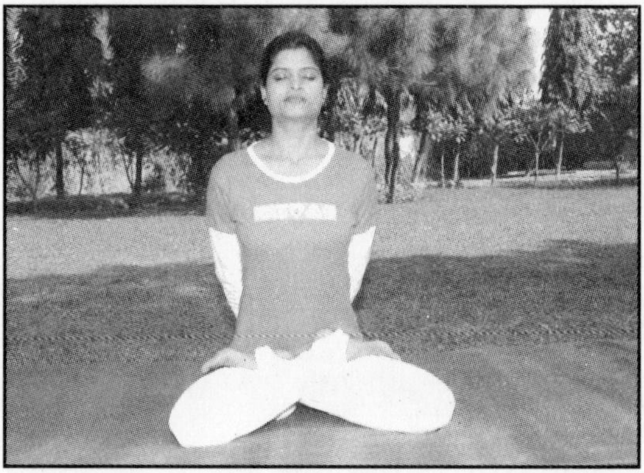

Yog Mudra Front View

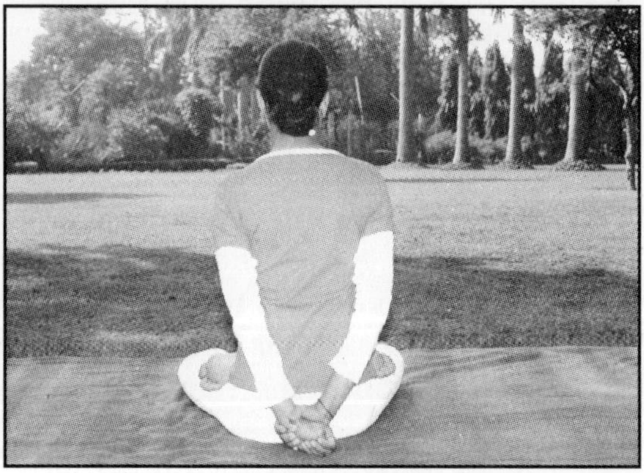

Yog Mudra Back View

Effects

This is a very useful asana for the spine, elbows, wrist, knees, ankles and hips. It also stimulates the gastric secretions, stimulates the production of bile, pancreatic juice and insulin. It also stimulates the adrenal glands and increases the production of corticosteroids (life-saving hormones).

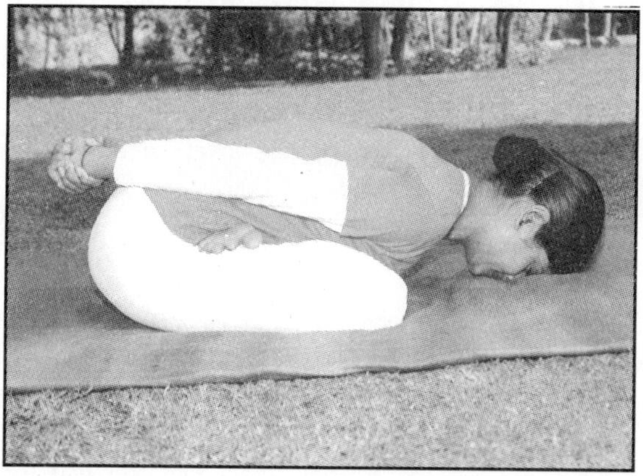

Yog Mudra (Right Side)

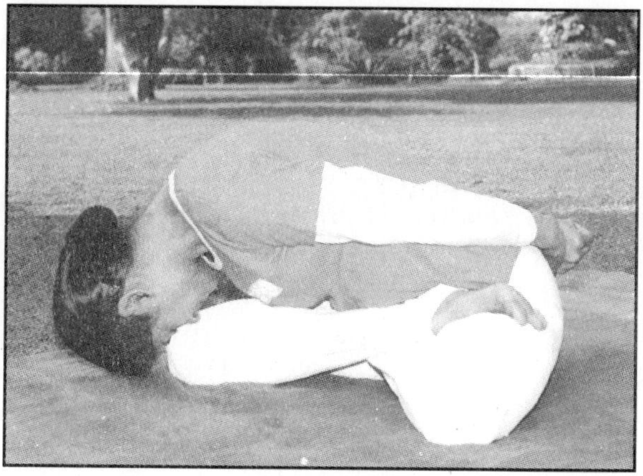

Yog Mudra (Left Side)

Caution

Yoga Mudra should not be attempted by:

(1) People suffering from arthritis of shoulders, elbows, wrists, hips, knees or ankles.

(2) By people with any deformity or dysfunction of the lumbar/ cervical spine.

(3) By people with deformed feet or hands.

(4) By people with chronic respiratory problems, particularly those who cannot hold the breath

Trikon Asana

This is performed in a standing position. Stand straight in the position of "Attention", with neck and body absolutely straight in one straight line. Open your feet, slightly more than the breadth of your shoulders. To concentrate on every act your eyes should remain closed while taking a long and deep breath, stretch your right arm outwards and gradually take it upwards till your right arm touches your right ear. Keep it fully stretched with the hand facing inwards and all the five fingers joined together. While exhaling (breathing out) bend your body from your lumber region towards the left side and try to touch the ground next to the left foot with your stretched left hand making sure that both the knees are absolutely straight and you are bending only sideways and not front ways, remain in this posture as long as it is comfortable, slowly come back to the upright position breathing in. Repeat the same procedure on the opposite side. This asana makes the spine flexible, exercises the muscles of the back, is helpful for the hip, knee, elbow and wrist joints, and is good for lungs as well as abdominal muscles.

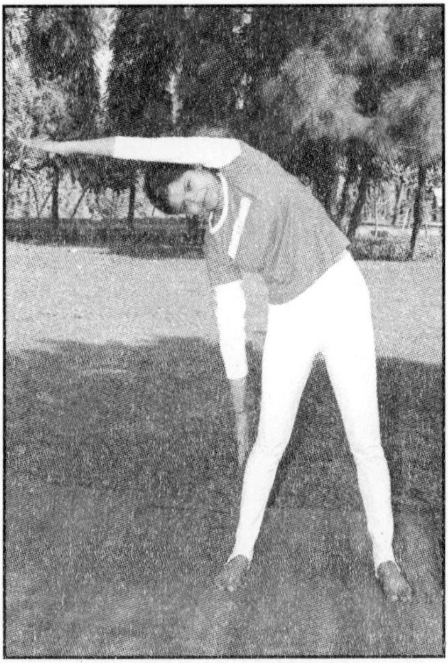

Trikon Asana (Left Stretch)

Effects

(1) It makes the spine flexible and pliable

(2) It is a good exercise for the side walls of chest and abdomen

(3) It exercises the muscles of legs as well as the arms

(4) It is also helpful in the mobility of the hip joint and the shoulder and ankle joints

Caution

It is difficult for people with weak chest and abdomen musculature to perform Trikon Asana. People with chronic respiratory problems should perform this asna with great caution.

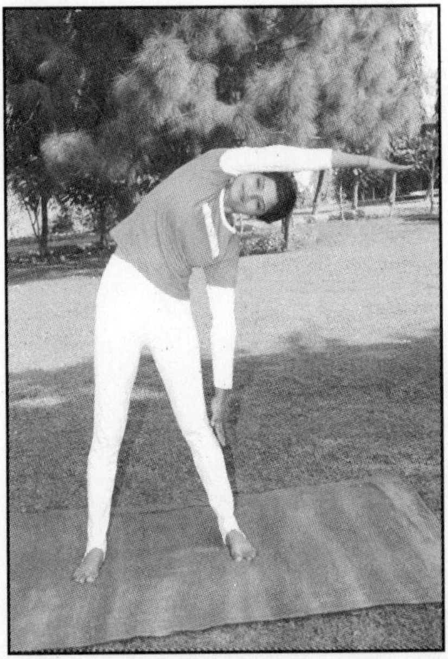

Trikon Asana (Right Stertch)

Body Stretch

This can be performed in standing as well as lying positions.

In standing position

Stand in the position of 'Attention' with both feet joined together. Stretch both arms above your head, intertwine the fingers of the left hand with the fingers of the right hand or keep the fingers straight and stretch both the shoulders upwards, keep them stretched. While taking a long and deep breath raise both the heels from the ground and try to stand on your toes, stretching both the shoulders as well as the lumber spine upwards. Maintain this position as long as it is comfortable and come back to the normal position while breathing out.

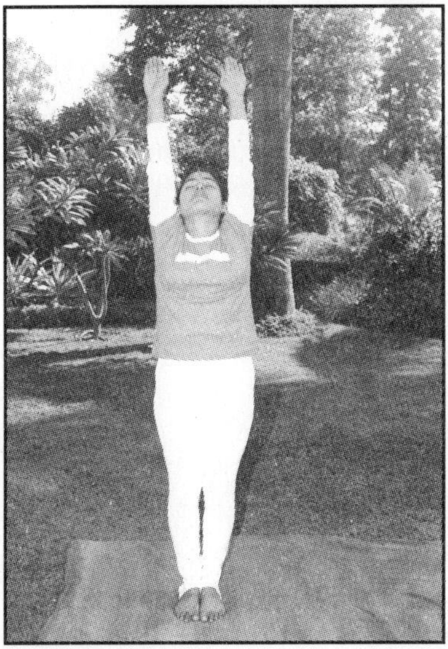

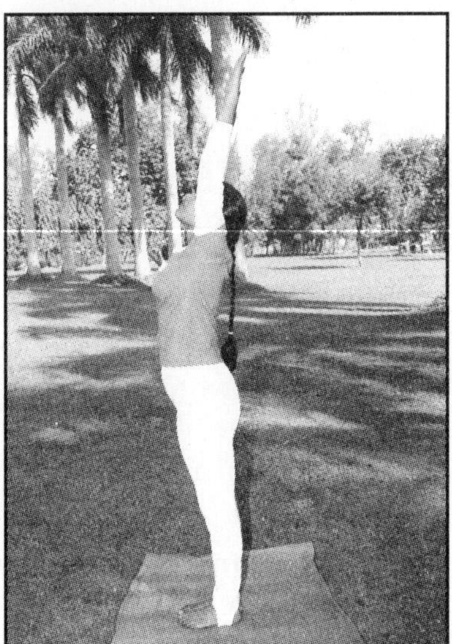

Body stretch (side view)

In lying position

Lie straight on your back with both the legs stretched and feet joined together, stretch your arms above your head making sure that the arms touch your respective ear. With your eyes shut concentrate on your belly button. While taking a long and deep breath, stretch the portion above the belly button upwards and the portion below the belly button downwards. Stretch as much as you can. When you find it uncomfortable gradually release your breath and come back to your normal position

Effects

This asana stretches most of the joints of the body including the spine, stretches most of the muscles of the body including the abdominal and back muscles and even stretches the viscera in chest as well as abdomen. One feels very fresh after this asana because this energises the whole body. Study the photographs carefully.

Camel Position (Usht Asana)

This is performed in a kneeling position. You stand on your bent knees; take your knees apart equal to the breadth of your shoulders or slightly more than that. Keep your back and neck straight. Keep both the thumbs at the back in the lumber region exactly behind the belly button, while the eight fingers of both the hands are fanned out and are pointing towards the belly button.

While pressing the thumbs forward and taking a deep breath, bend your back backwards leaving the neck loose so that the head hangs (see the photograph). Keep on bending this point backwards till you cannot go any further, stop here for a while. Take the hands away from the back and touch the palms with the respective sole. Take long and deep breaths. Maintain this position for a while. Now your spine is completely bent over like that of a camel and your head is still hanging backwards. Take a few deep breaths and revert to the upright position, still standing on your knees and supporting the back with your thumbs. Stay in this position for a while so that the blood circulation to the brain comes back to its normal position. Straighten your knees and go back to the resting position.

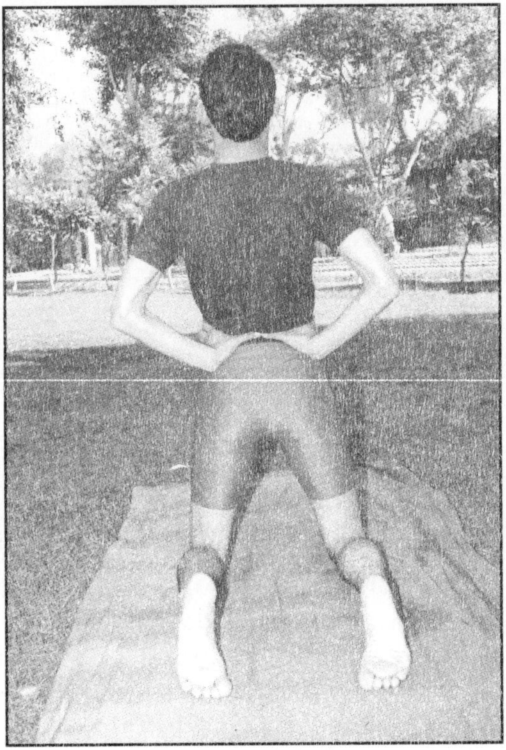

Camal Position (back view)

Effects

This is a very good asana for making the spine flexible. It strengthens the back muscles and is very good for lower backache. It also stretches the abdominal muscles and makes the stomach and intestines do their job properly. It also stimulates the glands in the abdomen.

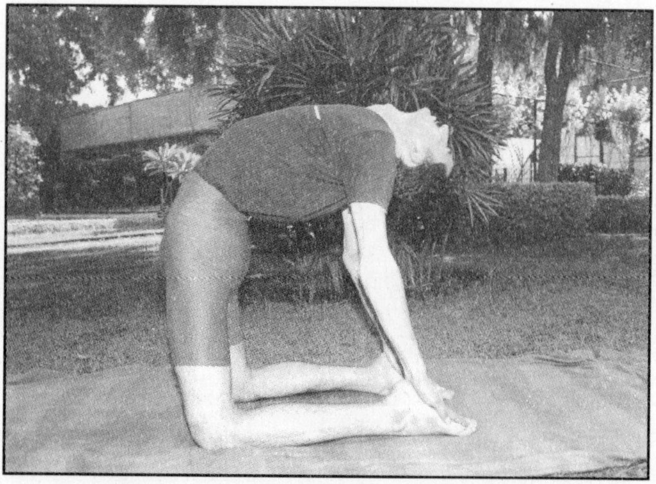

Camel Position (side view)

Caution

(1) People with bamboo spine cannot perform Usht Asana.

(2) It is difficult for people with arthritis of multiple joints, particularly knees, hips, spine, shoulders, elbows and wrist joints, to perform this asana.

(3) People with chest deformities will find it difficult to perform this asana.

Cobra Position (Bhujang Asana)

This is done in the lying position. Lie down on your tummy, keeping your legs stretched backward and your feet together. Touch your forehead with the ground keeping both the arms as close to the body as possible with elbows bent at ninety degrees and the hands facing the ground. Lift your head from the ground; touch the back of your head with the back of your chest. While breathing in gradually, slowly lift the front part of the body upwards. You have to lift the body with the help of the muscles of the back and spine. Try to lift the body up to your belly button; making sure that the whole weight is borne by the spine and not by the elbows or the hands. You have come to the cobra position, stay in the position as long as you can. Gradually start coming back to your original position by slowly breathing out, till your forehead touches the ground.

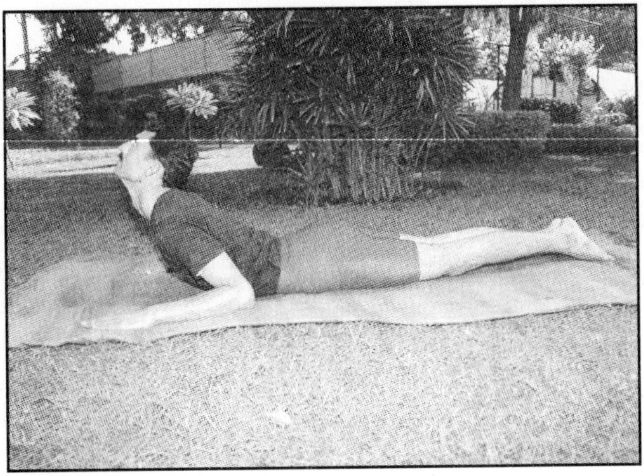

Cobra Position (side view)

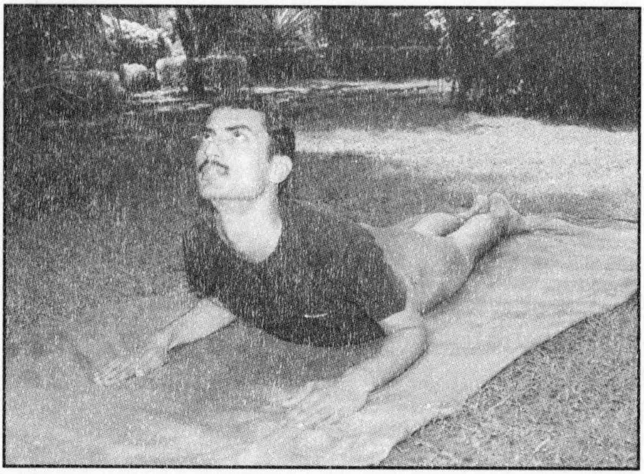

Cobra Position (front view)

Effects

This is an excellent asana for strengthening the upper and the middle back (cervical and dorsal regions) muscles. This stretches both the lungs, hence is a good exercise for the lungs, for the neck muscles and muscles of the chest.

This also energizes the Savadhishthana Chakra (refer to the chapter on Chakras), sending more energy to the sex organs.

Caution

(1) Any deformity/ arthritis of any portion of spine is a contraindication for performing this asana.
(2) People suffering from arthritis of shoulders, elbows or wrists perform this asna with difficulty.

Bow Position (Dhanur Asana)

This is also done in the lying position. You lie down on

your tummy with the forehead touching the ground in front and both feet joined together at the back. Bend both your knees; hold both the ankles with your respective hands. Take a deep breath, while breathing out lift both the knees from the ground (see the photographs).

Now while breathing in again lift the front part of the body backwards. Making your belly button as a fulcrum, your front as well as back is lifted up the ground; your back is curved forwards like a bow. Keep in this position as long as you can. While breathing out take back the knees to their original position and bring the forehead on to the ground and go to the resting position.

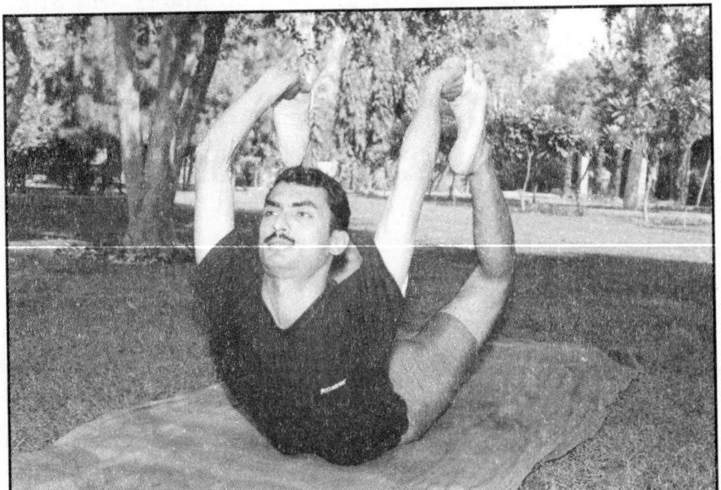

Bow Position (front view)

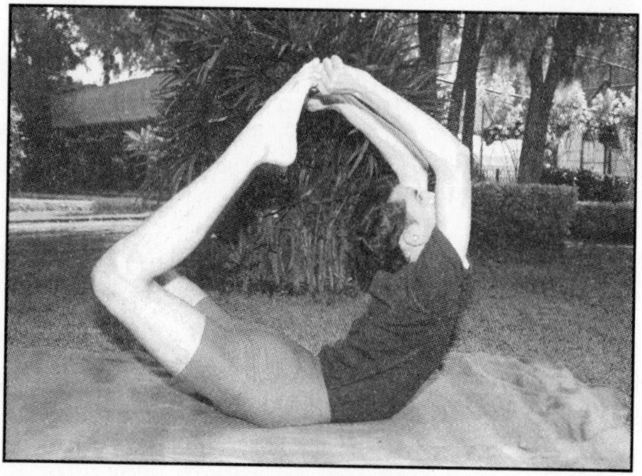

Bow Position (side view)

Effects

(1) Makes the spine flexible
(2) Strengthens the shoulders, knees and ankles
(3) Strengthens the chest muscles, shoulder muscles and back muscles
(4) It effects the abdominal organs as well as the ductless glands situated in the abdomen

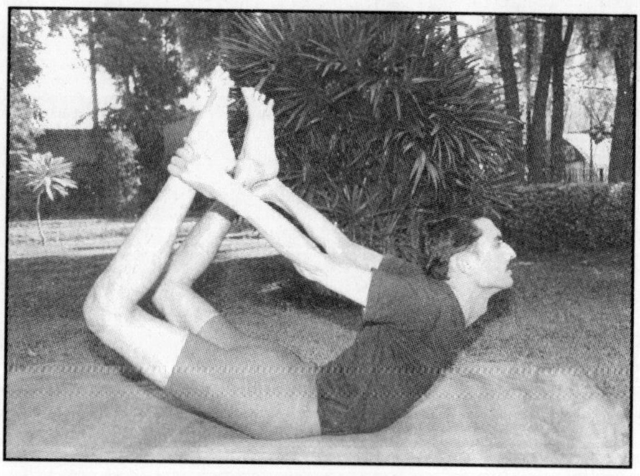

Bow Position (side view)

Caution

Arthritis or deformity of any portion of spine, of hips, knees, ankles, shoulder, elbows and wrists is a contraindication for performing this asana. This asana is also contraindicated in chronic chest problems.

Releasing the Wind from the Tummy (Pawan Mukt Asana)

This is done in the lying position. Lie on your back, keep both the legs straight with feet joined together. Bend the right knee, hold the bent knee with both the hands, and take a deep breath so that your tummy bulges out. Press the right knee with your tummy and keep on pressing. While keeping this pressed breathe out completely, raise your head and neck from the ground bend it forwards so that tip of the nose touches the right knee. Keep in this position as long as you can. While breathing out, bring your head back to its original position and then take your right knee back to its original position (refer to the photographs).

Repeat the same process on the left side while keeping your right knee straight and on the ground. Once you have finished with the left side, go back to your original position. Bend both the knee joints together, hold both the knees together with your hands, take a deep breath in, fill up your tummy, and press both the knees against the ballooned tummy. While breathing out, bring your head forwards and try to keep the tip of the nose in between the two knees. Breathe out completely, take the head back to its normal position, then take the knees back to their normal position and go to the resting position.

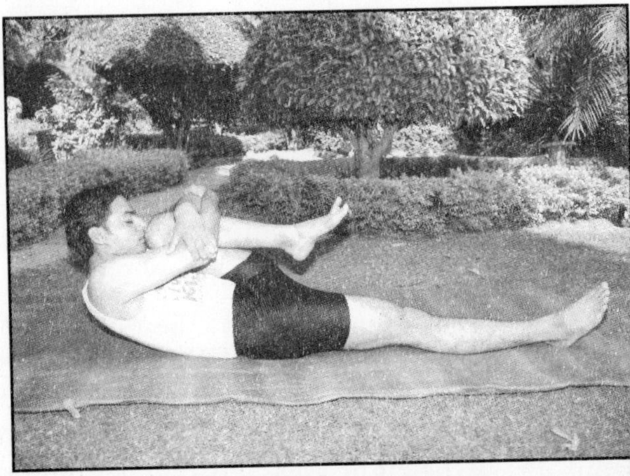

Pawan Mukt Asana with half knee bent

Effects

It is a very good asana for releasing wind from the tummy. It helps in digestion. It cures constipation. It is a very good exercise for the lungs as well as for the muscles of the back. It's a good exercise for both hips as well as knees.

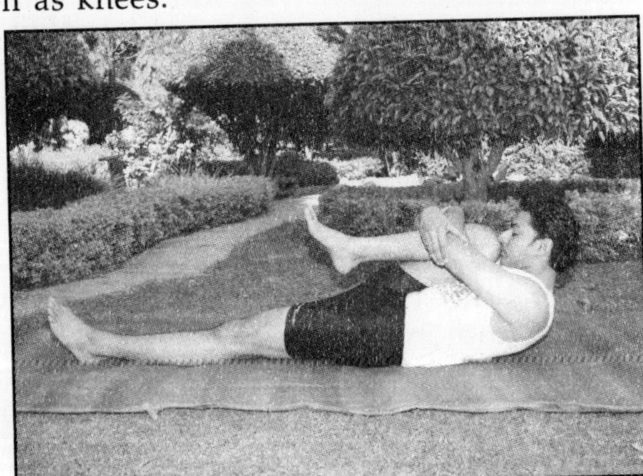

Pawan Mukt Asana with right knee bent

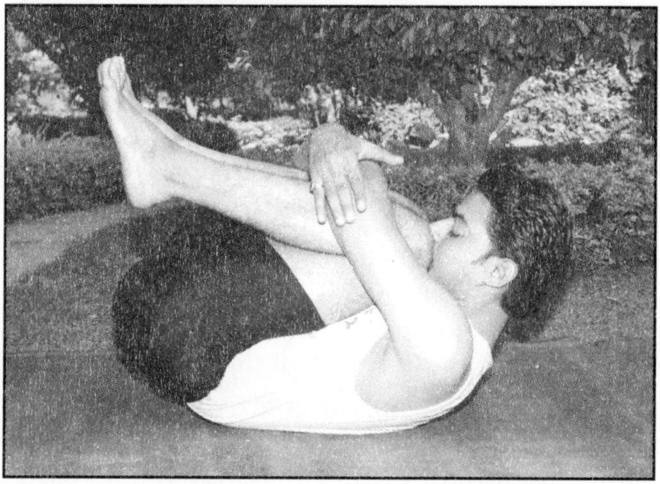

Pawan Mukt Asana with both knees bent

Caution

(1) People with arthritis of the knees, hips and wrist joints perform this asana with great difficulty.

(2) This asana should not be attempted by people suffering from chest deformities, chronic respiratory diseases and arthritis/ deformities of cervical spine.

Surya Parnam

Surya parnam means "salutation to the sun". This Asana has both physical as well as spiritual aspects. Yogic postures which provide exercise to all the parts of the body represent the physical aspects. Enjoyments derived by taking the blessing of the "Sun God" represent the spiritual side. The blessings asked for include progress in meditation, sound health, sharp mind and spiritual wisdom.

This asana should be performed with full attention and complete concentration. The sequence of this asana involves twelve body postures which represent twelve signs of the Zodiac through which passage of the sun results in the formation of twelve month of a year.

This asana involves six postures performing the exercise in one direction and six postures mark the return to the original position. The first six postures represent dakshinaayana (southerly course of the sun) for six months and returning six postures represent uttaraayana (northerly course of the sun) for six months.

All the twelve postures are synchronised with proper breathing *i.e.* inhalation, exhalation and pause. The most important part of this asana is recitation of proper mantras in proper manner, because this is the energy hidden in the mantra which is of significance.

This is an exclusive asana, which exercises all the joints of the body, all the muscles of the body, and all the systems of the body and energises the whole body. The twelve steps are:

Step 1 (Prayer with folded hands)

Stand erect, keeping both feet joined together, facing east. Make sure that your spine is absolutely straight and all the body muscles are in a tense state. Relax the whole body and fold both hands in front of the chest. The mantra for recitation is "Aum Mitraaya Namah" (salutation to the friend).

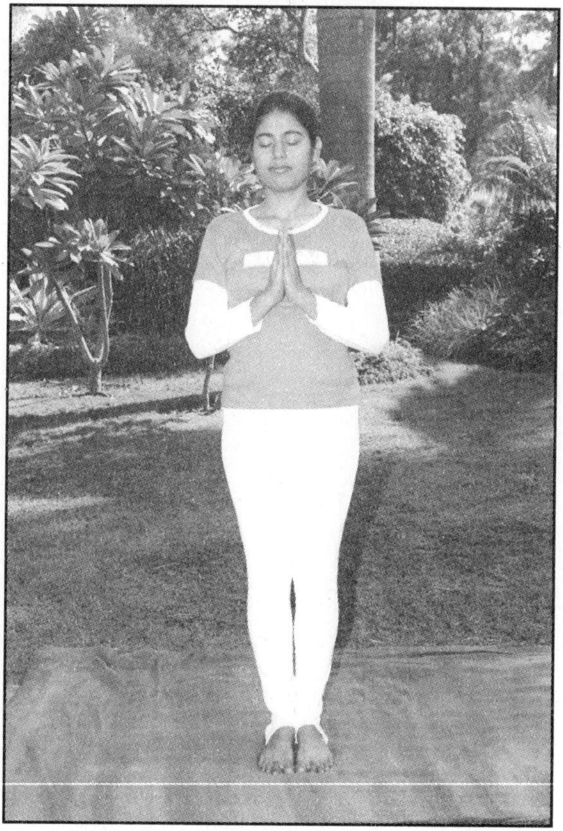

Surya Parnam Step 1

Step 2 (Prayer with raised arms)

While breathing in (inhaling) both the arms are raised above the head, completely stretch at the shoulder touching your ears. Carry the arms backwards along with the head extending the spine. The mantra for this step is "Aum Ravayai Namah" (Salutation to the effulgent one).

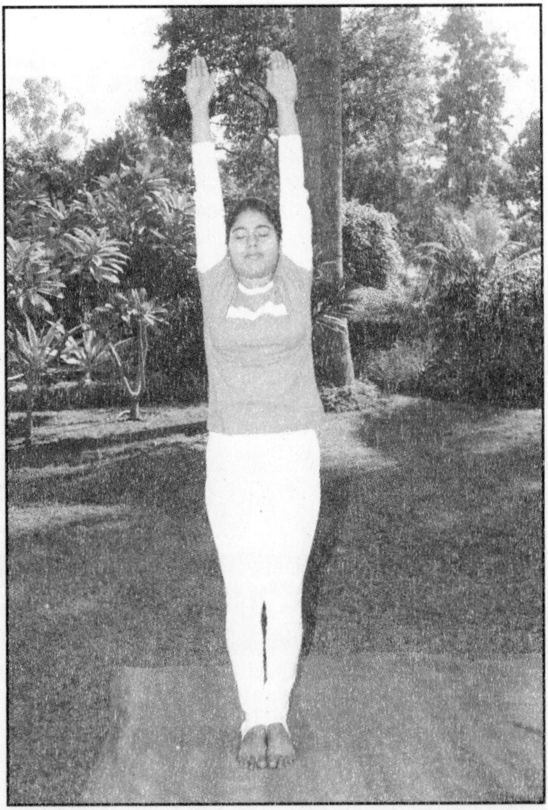

Surya Parnam Step 2

Step 3 (Forward bend)

Keeping the arms stretched at shoulders gradually bend forwards from the lumber spine while exhaling (breathing out). Place the palms of both hands on the ground on both sides of the feet so that all the ten fingers and ten toes are in a straight line. The knees should be kept straight, the abdomen should be completely empty and the chin should be touching the chest. The mantra for this step is:

"Aum Sooryaaya Namah" (Salutation to the luminous one).

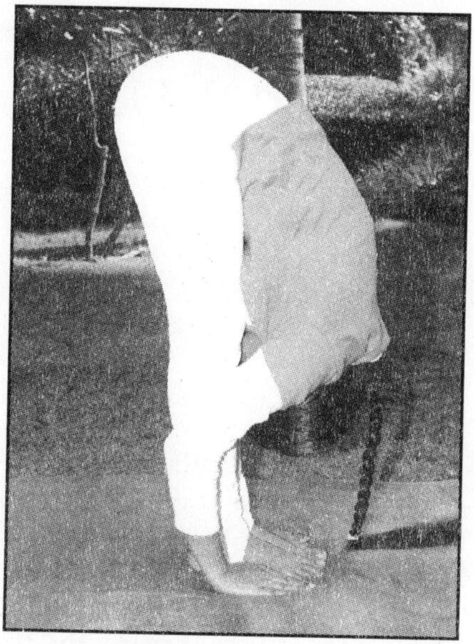

Surya Parnam Step 3

Step 4 (The horse position)

Keeping the hands where they are on the ground on either side of the feet, stretch the right leg backwards as far as you can making sure that the right knee touches the ground and the right foot is upright. The left knee is bent and left foot is placed formally on the ground. This whole process is done while breathing in (inhaling). The mantra for this step is:

"Aum Bhaanavae Namah" (Salutation to the brilliant one).

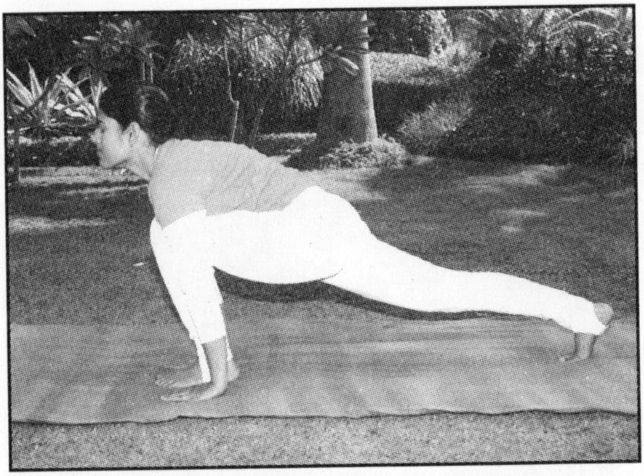

Surya Parnam Step 4

Step 5 (The Mountain)

While exhaling (breathing out) move the left foot backward so that both the feet are side by side to each other, lower the head and lift the back upwards making sure that your buttocks are as high up as possible. Keep both the legs as well as arms straight making sure that the soles of the two feet are formally on the ground and heels are touching each other. Mantra for this step is:

"Aum Khagaaya Namah" (Salutation to the one, moving in the sky).

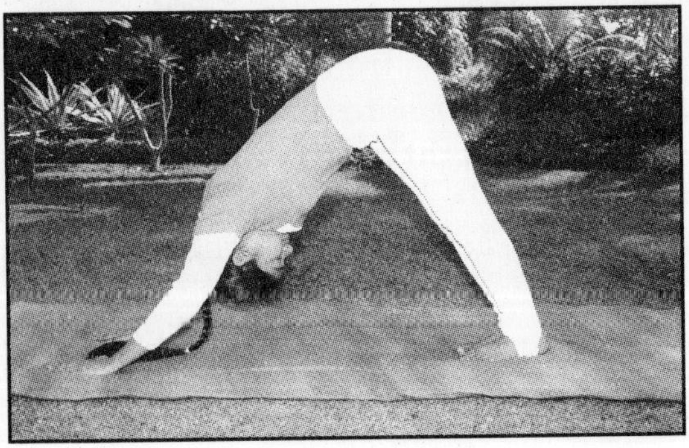

Surya Parnam Step 5

Step 6 (Salutation with eight points)

In this step eight body points are made to touch the ground. Lower the body and let the feet and knees touch the ground, keeping the feet in the upright position. Pull the abdominal muscles inward while lowering the chest and forehead to the ground, making sure that the hands are touching the ground and wrists are bent. In this position both feet, knees, chest, forehead and both hands are in contact with the ground while the hips and abdomen are lifted up from the ground. This step is preferably done while holding your breath outside the lungs. The mantra for this step is:

"Aum Pooshnae Namah" (Salutation to the giver of strength).

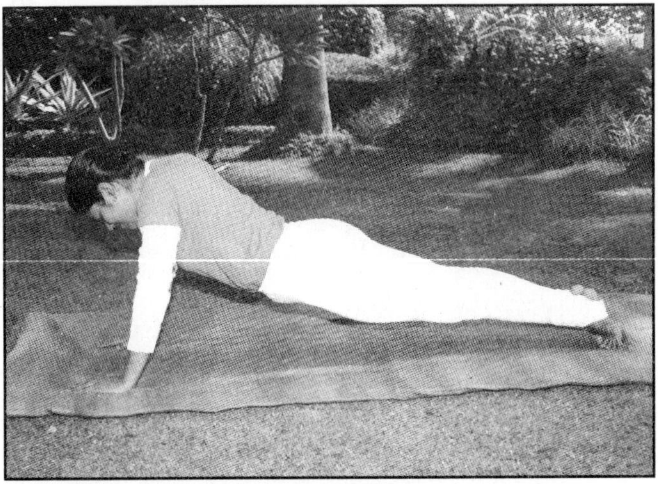

Surya Parnam Step 6

Step 7 (The Cobra)

From this step onward we gradually reverse six steps already performed. In this step straighten the arms at the elbows as well as shoulders keeping both the hands tightly with the ground while inhaling deeply, so that both the lungs are completely filled with the air. The spine and the head is bent backward so that front half of the body is raised from the ground and back half is formally touching the ground keeping the knees fully extended. The mantra for this step is;

"Aum Hiranyagarbhaaya Namah" (Salutation to the one, with the golden body).

Step 8 (The Mountain)

From this position come back to the mountain

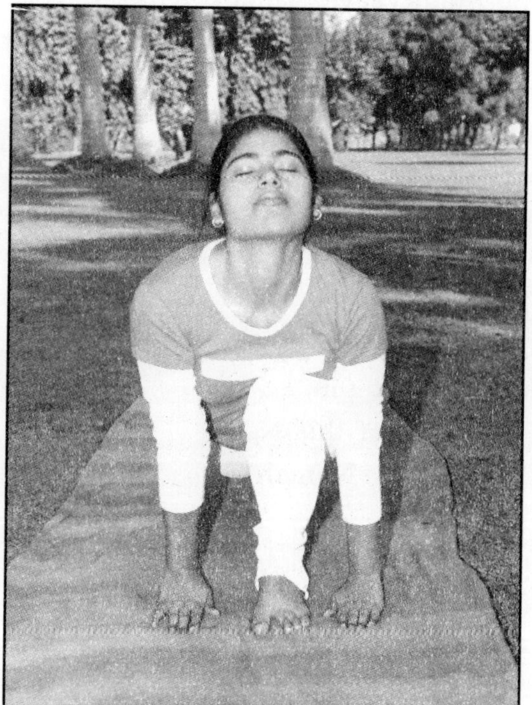

Surya Parnam Step 8

position already described in step 5, while breathing out (exhaling). The mantra for this step is:

"Aum Marichayae Namah" (Salutation to the lord of dawn).

Step 9 (The Horse)

In this step while inhaling deeply (breathing in) we go back to the horse position described in step 4 with the exception that in this step the right leg must be extended backwards and left leg brought forwards. The mantra for this step is:

"Aum Aadityaaye Namah" (Salutation to the son of Aditi)

Step 10 (Forward bend)

While breathing out (exhaling) we go back to the position described in step 3.

The mantra for this step is:

"Aum Savitrae Namah" (Salutation to the benevolent one).

Step 11 (Prayer with raised arms)

While breathing in, *i.e.* inhaling go back to step 2.

The mantra for this step is:

"Aum Arkaaya Namah" (Salutation to the shining one).

Step 12 (Prayer in standing position)

Return to the position in step 1 and breathe normally.

This is very important to synchronise physical postures with breathing. The appropriate mantras should be synchronised with postures as well as breathing. All the twelve steps are performed in one continuous sequence and rhythmic manner.

Effects

1. It is a complete asana in itself.
2. It exercises all the joints of the body, effects all the muscles of the body and influences all the ductless glands of the body.
3. It also energises all the seven major chakras.
4. It is a recommended technique to prepare the body for higher yogic practices, pranayam and meditation.
5. It removes emotional stress and makes a person calm and tranquil.

Caution

The people who have a healthy body and healthy system can perform this asana.

Resting Asanas

(1) Shav Asana

Shav asana is performed while lying on your back. Shav means dead body, hence it is exactly the way a dead body is lying with all the parts and all the group of muscles of the body completely relaxed, with both the feet apart by 30 to 45 centimetres. Both the arms lying along side the body with the fingers slightly flexed near the tips. Take regular deep breaths while watching your belly button. The belly button should rise up when you breathe in and should fall back when you breathe out. It is a state of complete relaxation, when we fill up the body with the fresh energy through the process of breathing (see the photographs).

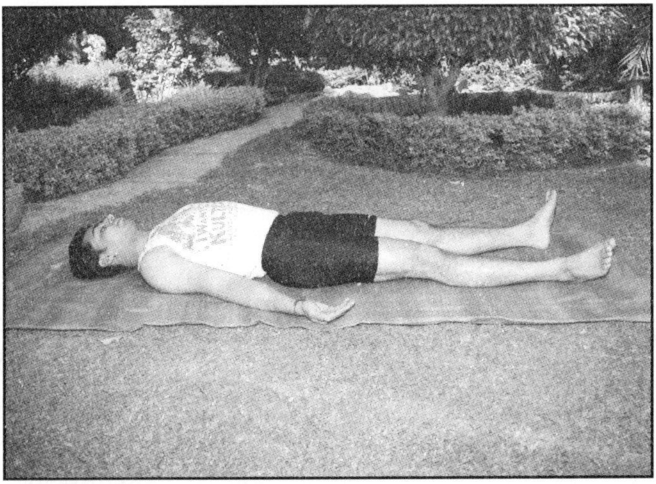

Shav Asana front side

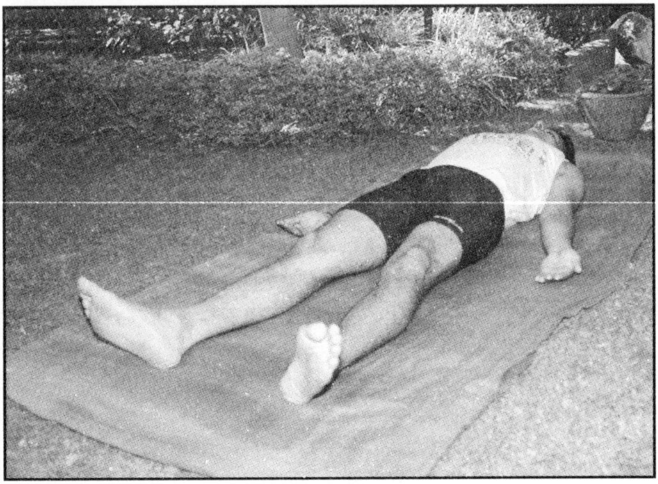

Shav Asana from front

(2) Sithal Asana

Resting either ear on the ground you may perform this asana. The steps being described are for the right ear resting on the ground.

Lie on your tummy making sure that both the lungs are resting on the ground; turn your face to the left side so that your right ear is touching the ground. Keep the right leg and right arm extended along the right side of the body with the palm of the right hand facing upwards towards the sky. Bend the left knee so that the left heel touches the right knee. The left arm is bent at the elbow with the palm of the hand facing the ground and all the five fingers joined together. This is exactly the position in which a baby sleeps. All the muscles of the body are completely relaxed and the eyes are closed, away from the distraction of the outside world. You take prolonged and deep breaths and set the mind to observe your breath. This is a state of complete relaxation, giving rise to bliss.

The same asana can be performed on the left ear, where everything is reversed (see the photograph).

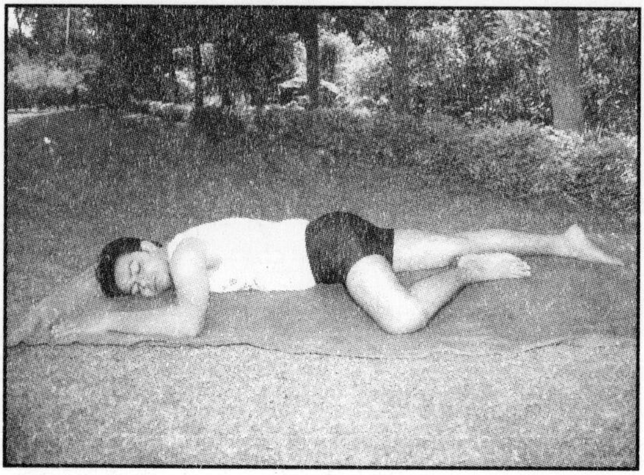

Sithal Asana in Right ear

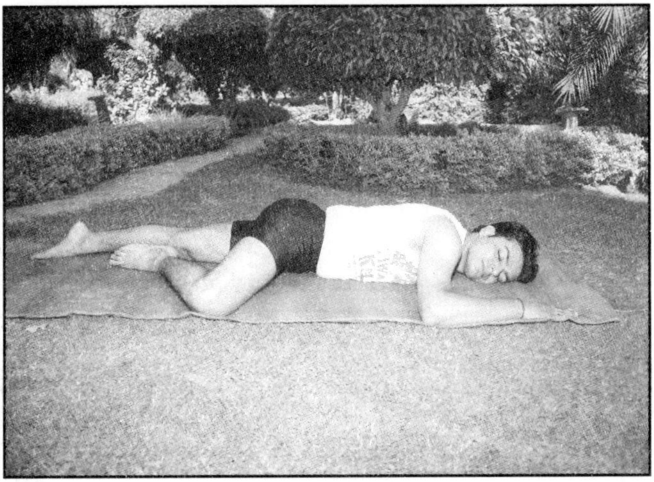

Sithal Asana in Left ear

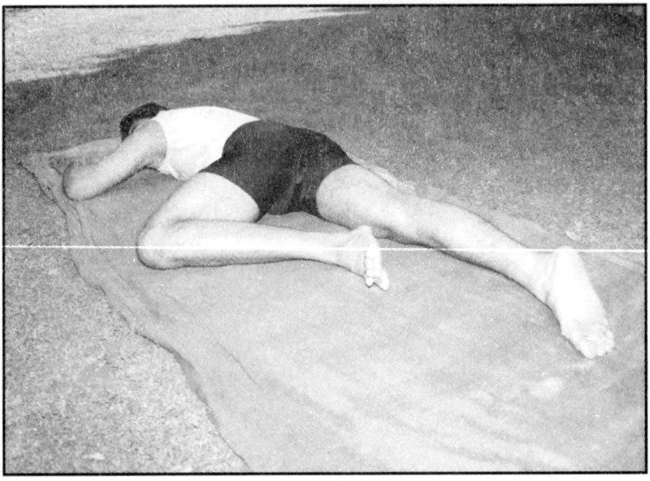

Sithal Asana (front view)

(3) Vishram position while sitting

Sit on your bottom with your arms placed on either side slightly behind your body. Extend the elbows,

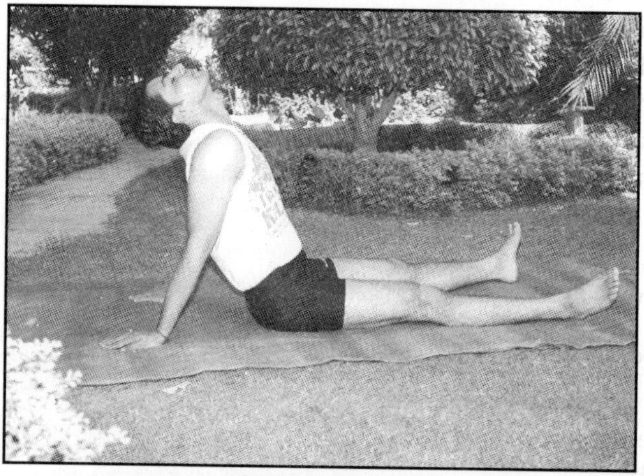

Vishram (side view)

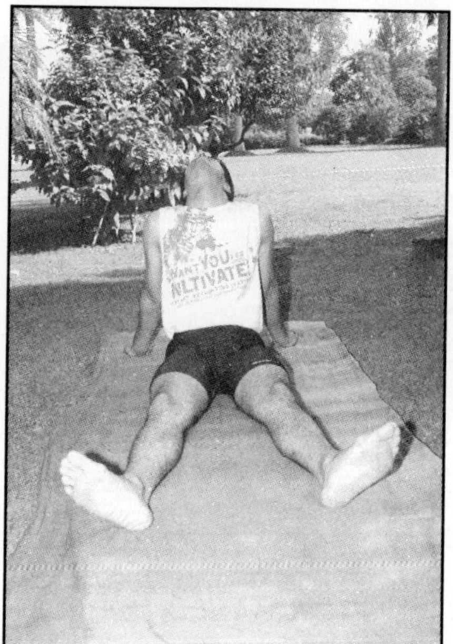

Vishram (front view)

palms pointing backwards and facing the ground. Both the legs are extended lying in front with both the back of the knees touching the ground; feet are kept apart by 30 to 45 centimetres. The spine is reclining backwards slightly and the neck is hanging loose with the eyes closed.

In all the resting exercises deep and prolonged breathing plays a very important part in re-energising the whole body (see the photograph).

Effects of resting asanas

All the resting asanas are meant to energise the different parts of the body to bring the rhythm back to the breathing, to calm the nerves and the mind. Shav Asana has been found very helpful in bringing the high blood pressure down.

Caution

There is hardly any caution for performing Shav Asana but people suffering from arthritis of the knees, elbows and wrists might find it difficult to perform Sithal Asana and Vishram Asana in the resting position.

Asanas for strengthening the Pelvic Floor

Pelvic floor is formed by a group of muscles, which are not visible to our eyes but play a vital role in maintaining our life, particularly the sex life. This also plays a vital role in women during childbirth. Pelvic floor forms the floor of the abdomen, whereas diaphragm forms the roof of the abdomen. The layers of muscles, which lie within the pelvic walls, form the pelvic floor. Pelvic floor is pierced by two very important openings *i.e.* the back passage (anus) which facilitates the passage of stools and the front passage (Urethra) which facilitates the passage of urine. In women there is a third opening below the front passage called the vagina. Special muscle fibers form sphincters, which guard all these three openings. If one sphincter is made to contract, then all the three sphincters contract. Anal sphincter usually remains in a state of full contraction except when you are emptying your bowels whereas urethral and vaginal sphincters are normally in a state of partial contraction. All the three sphincters can be contracted or relaxed whenever we desire (are under our conscious control).

For strengthening the pelvic muscle, the following asanas are recommended.

(1) Squatting position

This may be done without any support by squatting on the ground/ floor or may be done sitting on a low stool or squatting against a wall, squatting with support under the heels or full squatting while standing.

Procedure

While squatting you sit with both knees bent, feet firmly on the ground and the pelvic diaphragm is not supported.

When you begin the process of squatting breathe in (inhale) and holds your breath while squatting, gradually breathe out (exhale) while standing up.

This is an excellent exercise for strengthening the pelvic floor muscles; you may also relax any of your sphincters, which you wish to relax.

(2) Forward bend

Step 1: Keep your feet apart equal to the distance between your shoulders.

Step 2: Bend forwards keeping your knees straight.

Step 3: Place both your palms on the ground in front while keeping your elbows extended.

The body weight is borne by both the feet as well as the hands. The pelvic muscles are stretched and so are the muscles of the thigh and calf.

Moola Bandha

For the detailed procedure for Mool bandha see under the heading of Bandhas.

Effects

Although Mool bandha is primarily used for contracting and pulling up the anal canal, but, as mentioned earlier, if one sphincter contracts the others automatically contract because they are all part of one muscle. Hence Mool bandha is a very good exercise for all the three sphincters *i.e.* anal sphincter, urethral sphincter and vaginal sphincter. Exercise of these sphincters is essential because when it comes to relaxing a sphincter the other sphincters should remain contracted. During the process of urination we do not wish to pass stools, hence the urethral sphincter is relaxed whereas the anal sphincter remains contracted.

In women, during love-making the vaginal sphincter will contract and relax whereas the anal as well as the urethral sphincters shall remain contracted.

Effects of strengthening pelvic floor

Strengthening and exercising the pelvic floor helps the following:

(1) In the sphincter control of the urinary bladder and anus.

(2) In the process of love making, helping in rhythmic contraction of vaginal muscles.
(3) Very helpful during the birth of a baby, when a woman has to bear down during the pains to expel the baby.
(4) Very helpful for strengthening the pelvic floor after the birth of the baby.
(5) Helpful in retaining the pelvic organs in their respective position.
(6) Helpful in stimulating the secretions of testes in males and ovaries in females.

Systematic Control of the Breath (Pranayam)

3

Systematic Control of the Breath (Pranayam)

Pranayam is a Sanskrit word, 'Pran' means Vital Energy, which we obtain in the form of atmospheric oxygen through the process of breathing. 'Yam' means regulation. Regulation of breath is called 'Pranayam'.

Pranayam is based on the principle of filling the lungs with maximum amount of atmospheric oxygen, keeping that oxygen for a sufficient length of time in the lungs to allow for gaseous exchange to take place between the blood and inhaled breath. Blood well saturated with oxygen can impart a better quality of energy to different tissues of the body.

Pranayam also brings a proper rhythm to the breathing. Breathing connects us to the earth as well as the cosmos and generates the power to bring mind, body, spirit and emotions in harmony.

To understand the process involved in different pranayams it is essential to understand the process of normal breathing.

Normal Breathing

Normal breathing involves breathing the atmospheric

air into the lungs (*inhaling*), keeping it there for a while (*pause*, this is called *Kumbak* in Sanskrit) and breathing out (*exhaling*).

For this process to take place fully certain tissues, muscles, organs come into play.

One can breathe either through the mouth or through the nose. People who breathe through the mouth are called mouth breathers whereas those who breathe through their nose are called nose breathers. There is an advantage to breathing through the nose.

Advantages of breathing through the nose

(1) It is a noiseless process.

(2) Hairs inside the nose act as filters for the bacteria and suspended particles in the atmospheric air.

(3) While passing through the nose the temperature of the inhaled air is adjusted with the body temperature of the individual.

(4) While passing through the nose the dry atmospheric air becomes moist, because of the secretion of the nose.

(5) Breathing through the nose helps in replacing the air in the sinuses with the fresh air, which in turn sends more oxygen to the brain through the process of diffusion.

(6) Nasal breathing stimulates olfactory bulbs in the brain, which in turn makes breathing rhythmic.

Disadvantages of breathing through the mouth

(1) Breathing through the mouth always produces a little croupy noise.

(2) Mouth breathers are always heavy breathers.

(3) Breathing through the mouth makes the mouth dry causing uneasiness and discomfort. It also disrupts the normal functioning of various tissues in the mouth like the tongue and mucus membranes.

(4) Breathing through the mouth disrupts the sound box leading to a peculiar noise, which during sleep produces 'snoring'.

(5) Breathing through the mouth does not allow the inhaled air to get adjusted to the body temperature.

(6) Mouth breathers develop prominent and defective teeth in the upper jaw, which gives their mouth a peculiar shape.

From the nose or the mouth the breathed air passes into the wind pipe called the '*Trachea*', which is located in the front of the neck. As soon as the trachea enters the chest it divides into two parts, the right part called the right bronchus goes to the right lung. The left part called the left bronchus goes to the left lung.

Lungs

There are two lungs, which are placed in the chest. The left lung is smaller than the right lung because it provides space for the heart. The lungs resemble a sponge and their ultimate unit is called an 'air sac'. An *air sac* is a balloon like structure, which is filled with the atmospheric air and on the other side of the sac runs the blood. There is a single celled wall separating the air from the blood where gaseous exchange takes place between the air and the blood by the process of diffusion. In this process atmospheric oxygen is taken up by the blood and carbon dioxide, water vapor and other waste products are released by the blood into the air, which is thrown out into the atmosphere by the process of 'exhalation'. There are millions of air sacs in each lung where this process takes place. The process of diffusion of gases is more complete if the inhaled air is allowed to stay in the lungs for a longer time.

In front, long flat bones called 'ribs', protect the lungs. There are twelve pairs of ribs *i.e.* twelve ribs on the right side of the chest and twelve ribs on the left side of the chest. These ribs are connected to each other by muscles called intercostal muscles. At the back, the lungs are again supported by the back portion of the twelve ribs on each side along with the backbone and back intercostal muscles. Ribs and intercostal muscles play a very important part in the process of breathing. Intercostal muscles are also called muscles for breathing.

Another important muscle, which separates the chest from the abdomen (belly), is called the diaphragm.

Diaphragm

This is a dome (tent) shaped flat muscular sheet, which separates the chest from the abdomen. It has a very important function to play in the process of breathing because under normal circumstances the bases of both the lungs are placed on the dome of this muscle.

When we breathe in (inhale) the lungs expand and the area of the chest increases. The bases of the lungs push the dome of the diaphragm downwards, which becomes flat, increasing the intra abdominal pressure. When we breathe out the lungs contract, the diaphragm rises up, increasing the pressure in the chest, which in turn throws the air out from the lungs. Hence, inhaling is a passive process whereas exhaling is an active process.

Breathing process gives rise to rhythmic movement of the diaphragm which in turn massages the organs lying above as well as below it and stimulate them to perform their functions in a normal healthy manner. In other words, rhythmic breathing influences the blood circulation, process of digestion and insulin production.

The diaphragm plays a very important role in certain pranayams.

Process of normal breathing

We breathe the atmospheric air through our nose/ mouth into our lungs. This process of breathing in, is called *inhalation*, which is followed by a *pause*. During this pause the gaseous exchange takes place between the breathed in air and the blood, which is followed by breathing the air out. This process is called *exhalation*. This is again followed by a pause and we start the next cycle of breathing the air in.

Inhalation ⟶ Internal Pause ⟶ Exhalation ⟶ External Pause ⟶ Inhalation

This cycle of breathing starts at the time of birth and continues till the time of death. A normal person breathes 15 to 18 times a minute. This is increased if the person is emotionally upset or mentally tense. One can have voluntary control over one's breath but only to some extent.

The vital component in the air which provides energy to each and every cell/tissue of the body is oxygen, but modern research shows that there is something else in the air, which also gives vital energy to the body. No definite name has been given to this but it may be called as 'prana', in Sanskrit or 'Chi' in Chinese.

Air is called pure if it has higher concentration of oxygen whereas impure air besides having low concentration of oxygen has higher concentration of carbon dioxide, nitrogen and other waste products.

Polluted air has a lower concentration of oxygen, a higher concentration of carbon dioxide, nitrogen, sulphur dioxide, other poisonous gases and suspended particles including bacteria and viruses etc.

PRANAYAM

Purpose of pranayam

The purpose of pranayam is:

- To regulate breathing.
- To inhale as much air as possible, to increase the depth of breathing.
- To increase the pause after inhaling, to allow sufficient time for gaseous exchange to take place.
- To exhale completely to empty all the air sacs, so that all the old/dead air is thrown out.

Pre-requisites for performing pranayam

(1) Pranayam can be performed at any time of the day, but it should preferably be performed when atmosphere is laden with fresh oxygen.

Early in the morning when the light rays fall on the trees, oxygen is released in abundance, the temperature of the atmosphere is cool, and this is the best time for performing pranayam.

Pranayam may also be performed at the end of the day when the sun is going to set. The atmosphere again has comparatively more concentration of oxygen and the atmospheric temperature has also started coming down.

(2) It is essential to have healthy nasal passages and healthy breathing apparatus for performing pranayam.

(3) It is essential to have a healthy and clean mind with positive thinking, which can concentrate with every act of breathing.

(4) It is advisable to evacuate your bowels and bladder before starting pranayam.

(5) Pranayam should preferably be performed on an empty stomach.

(6) Hatha Yoga recommends that pranayam should be practised four times a day *i.e.* early in the morning, noon, evening and before going to bed. This regimen is very difficult to follow in the modern day and age.

(7) Pranayam should be performed at a place where there is plenty of fresh air *i.e.* in the open and not in a closed room.

(8) Pranayam should be performed with determination and regularity.

(9) Pranayam should always be performed through the nose and never through the mouth.

Procedure for pranayam

(1) Pranayam is best performed in an upright sitting position, to allow energy to run up and down the spine and invigorate the different Chakras. The best position is the lotus position. But pranayam can be performed in any other posture *i.e.* while sitting on a chair, reclining, lying down on your back and even in the standing position.

(2) All the body muscles should be fully relaxed, particularly the muscles of the face with a light smile on the face. With the passage of time a glow appears on the face of those people who perform pranayam regularly.

(3) The eyes should always be kept closed while performing pranayam, so that the senses do not get distracted outwardly. It allows the mind to concentrate on each and every act of pranayam without which the pranayam is not effective.

(4) It is preferable to keep the tongue held with the palate, because it helps the mind to concentrate and does not allow the saliva to accumulate in the mouth.

(5) During the process of inhalation the chest should expand, the tummy should come forward and the belly button should become prominent. During the process of exhalation the chest should contract, tummy along with the belly button should go back and preferably touch the backbone. The pause should be reasonable.

(6) The head should hang down slightly and chin should rest in between the two collarbones.

(7) The left arm is kept straight and the left wrist is resting on the left knee, the index finger is touching the tip of the thumb and the other three fingers are extended facing upwards (Gyan Mudra). This posture is required where the right hand is used for blocking the one or the other nostril.

(8) Never try to exceed your body capacity in performance of pranayam. With practice you will be able to increase the timing for each act of pranayam.

(9) It is preferable to perform pranayam after yoga asanas, but a reasonable amount of time must elapse between the last asana and pranayam so as to allow the body and breath to come to its normal position and rhythm.

(10) Try to achieve an even ratio in inhalation and exhalation. In the beginning the time spent for inhalation should be equal to the time spent on exhalation.

(11) It is essential to learn to increase the time of pause between inhalation and exhalation. It sometimes needs long practice to learn the process of pause rhythmically.

Do's & Don'ts for pranayam

(1) Pranayam should not be performed by sick people.

(2) Pranayam should be performed very carefully and under supervision if one is suffering from

chronic respiratory disease or chronic nasal disease.

(3) Pranayam should be performed very carefully during pregnancy. Certain pranayams are absolutely prohibited during pregnancy.

(4) People suffering from heart disease, high blood pressure, chronic lung disease, Glaucoma (kala motia), chronic Supportive otitis media (pus in the ears) should not attempt to have an unduly long pause between inhalation and exhalation.

(5) While doing pranayam you should never exceed your body limits.

Effects of pranayam

(1) Pranayam clears the nasal passages and helps in keeping them as well as the sinuses in a healthy state.

(2) Pranayam energises and vibrates the brain cells helping to improve the memory.

(3) Pranayam is a source of fresh and new energy to all energy channels (nadis) in the body.

(4) Pranayam not only helps in regulating the breath but also helps in stabilising the mind and the thought process, in turn increasing the concentration of the mind.

(5) Pranayam helps in calming down the senses and sensory impulses and tries to chanellise the senses to divert the energy, which runs after the outside worldly objects to look inside and utilise that energy for spiritualisation. Craving of the senses for worldly pleasure,

which one derives from smoking, drinking and by excessive indulgence in sex is also reduced.

6. Pranayam helps in cooling down the temperament
7. Pranayam connects you to the cosmos when you inhale and connects you with the earth and its gravity when you exhale.
8. Pranayam ultimately leads to the process of meditation, dhyana and even Samadhi.

Explanation of Yogic Prana and Bandhas

I do not intend to write a detailed book on pranayam, but I do wish to mention certain important procedures. By performing these procedures on a daily basis the readers can get tremendous benefits and keep their body systems in good health and shape.

Before I embark upon explaining techniques of different pranayams, it is essential to explain prana and bandhas.

Yogic prana (vital energy)

In yoga energy has been divided into ten different components, which perform different vital functions. These are *prana, apana, samana, udana, vyana, naga, kurma, krikla, devaditta* and *dhananjaya.* Out of these prana and apana are most important.

Prana

The atmospheric air, which we breathe in and out, has been given the name of prana in yoga, because it contains oxygen which is vital for the function of all the body tissues. It is also said that there is something else which gives energy to the body (but it has not been clearly defined so far) and that is called prana. This is that vital energy (air) which moves in the region of the heart. Prana energy is said to move upwards.

Apana

This is that part of vital energy which moves downwards and has its seat in the anus, which helps in the movement of the stools downwards, hence relieving constipation and helping in the process of defecation. The movement of air is in the region of the lower abdomen.

(For better understanding of all the vital airs the reader is referred to the book called *Vital Energy* by the same author.)

With this much understanding of the prana (vital air), we shall now proceed to explain Bandhas, because they form an important part of the whole system of pranayam.

BANDHAS (LOCKS)

The singular for Bandhas is Bandh which means blocking or putting a stop to something to regulate it. Here we stop the breath at different levels to regulate the energy to particular parts of the body. Bandhas are practised for stabilising the prana and for their retention in the body for a longer duration. Basically, there are three Bandhas called (1) Jalandhar Bandh, (2) Uddiyan Bandh, and (3) Mool Bandh.

Jalandhar Bandha

Jala means a "web" or a mesh.

Procedure

In Jalandhar Bandha throat and neck are contracted, so that chin touches the upper part of the chest. The chin rests on the notch between the two collar bones, which regulates the flow of prana and blood to the heart, thyroid gland and the region of the head and neck which includes the *brain*. During Jalandhar Bandha less blood rushes towards the heart, eyes and ears creating a feeling of giddiness and imbalance in the body.

Jalandhar Bandha helps in regulation of all three components of breathing *i.e.* inhalation, exhalation and retention of breath.

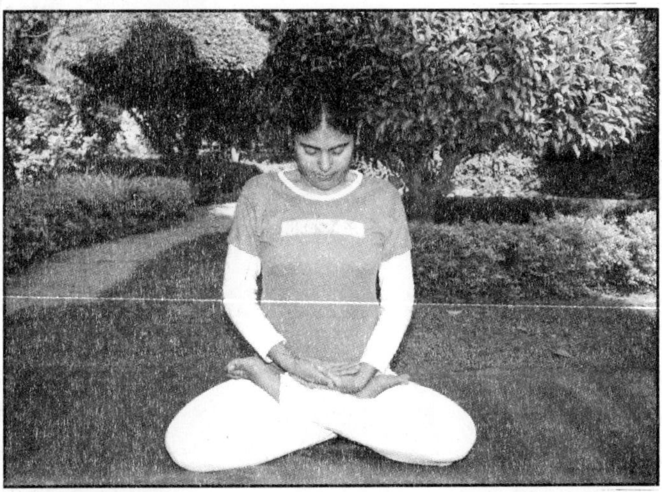

UDDIYANA BANDHA

Uddiyana means to lift. In this bandha we lift the diaphragm (a tent-like muscle separating the chest from abdomen) high up in the thorax (chest), which pulls the organs lying in the upper part of the abdomen like esophagus and stomach upwards against the spine.

Procedure

Uddiyana Bandha is performed by exhaling completely and during the external pause, by sucking the abdominal muscles and belly button inwards and backwards towards the spine.

Uddiyana Bandha forces the Prana to enter into "Sushmana Nadi". Sushmana Nadi is the main channel which carries the flow of nervous energy and is situated in the centre of the spinal cord.

This Bandha helps in energising the tent-like muscle called diaphragm, upper abdominal organs and abdominal muscles. It also gives a gentle massage to the heart muscle.

Improperly performed Uddiyana Bandha causes involuntary discharge of semen and loss of vital fluid.

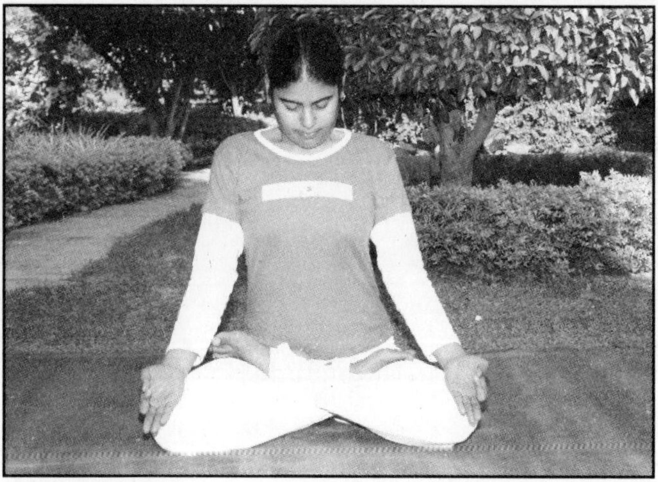

MOOLA BANDHA

Mool means root, origin or foundation.

Procedure

Moola Bandha is performed by contracting the part of the pelvic diaphragm upwards between anus and scrotum in males and between anus and vagina in females. By contracting this region, Apana *i.e.* energy in the lower abdomen, which normally takes downward course is made to flow upwards to unite with prana which has its seat in the chest region.

Moola Bandha should be performed during the retention of the breath. It can be performed during external as well as internal retention. During retention of the breath, the anus is pulled upwards towards the belly button against the spine. This creates a pull on pelvic diaphragm as well as diaphragm muscle separating the chest and abdomen. The entire region from anus to diaphragm is pulled up towards the spine.

This Bandha tones up the perennial muscles and pelvic organs, which include prostrate, bladder, vaginal muscles and uterine muscles (in females), by doing so it helps in the enjoyment during conjugal relations by increasing the sexual power.

Improperly performed Moola Bandha, leads to weakness of the body and lack of virility.

It is said that by performing all these Bandhas regularly, twenty-one vital parts of the body are rejuvenated. These parts include:

2 thumbs

2 ankles

2 knees

2 hips

2 middle of the eyebrows
1 prepuce
1 organs of generation
1 navel (belly button)
1 heart
1 neck
1 throat
1 palate
1 nose
1 forehead
1 head
1 crown aperture

Regular and proper performance of Bandhas generates more sexual and sensual energies. If a yogi directs these energies downwards and outwards, he enjoys sensual pleasure, but if he directs these energies upwards and inwards he enjoys the 'Bliss' and 'Nirvana'. It is said that when sexual energy is directed upwards, it becomes 'Oja' or energy for enlightenment. Practice of Mool Bandha makes one reach the only and true source of creation and helps in winning over the 'Ego'.

Jalandhar Bandha helps in stabilising the prana air and its retention for a longer period. Moola Bandha stabilises the apana air which has a tendency to move downwards. Moola bandha also helps in uniting the prana and apana airs. Uddiyana Bandh helps in the movements of the united prana, apana air to assend upwards. We shall describe the process and functions of these three Bandhas separately.

Moola Bandha

This is called Mool bandh because it is practised at the root of the spine by contracting the anal sphincter and drawing the rectum upwards, which helps in the movement of the *'apana'* air upwards (the normal tendency of the apana air is to move downwards). This way the "apana air" is allowed to unite with the *"prana air"* and this united prana-apana air is made to enter into the sushmana nadi (for description of this nadi see the chapter on energy).

Moola bandha can be practised in any position i.e. sitting, lying, standing, walking, and sitting on a chair or while performing any task.

Effects of Moola Bandha

1. It tones up the intestinal system.
2. It tones up the pelvic organs including sex organs and excretory system.
3. It refines the sexual desires.
4. It stimulates all the three lower chakras. Stimulation of the Manipura chakra increases the digestive power.
5. It helps in controlling the breath by soothing the nerves.
6. Moola bandha is used very frequently during different processes of pranayam.

Uddiyana Bandha

There are 72 thousand nadis, which cross, form clusters or criss-cross at the navel (belly button) region. Uddiyana bandha activates the navel region, hence energises the whole network of the nadis in the body. It also helps in guiding the prana into the sushmana nadi.

While performing Uddiyana Bandha the lungs are completely emptied by a forceful exhalation followed by contraction of the abdominal muscles, which will draw the navel (belly button) towards the backbone so that the root of the naval rests against the backbone.

Effects of Uddiyana Bandha

1. The most important effect of Uddiyana Bandha is that it allows the united prana-apana air enter in the Brahm nadi (sushmana nadi), which gives refreshing and soothing energy to the upper parts of the body. This function can only be performed properly if Uddiyana Bandha is applied in conjunction with Moola Bandha
2. This bandha is very helpful in "Agnisar Pranayam", which is described in subsequent pages.
3. It strengthens the abdominal muscles and the muscles of the intestines, hence helping the contractility of the intestines, which results in pushing the waste products into the intestines downward towards the rectum.
4. In yoga it is thought that sexual energy moves in the same direction in which the prana moves (normally sex energy moves downwards). Since in Uddiyan bandh the prana energy is moving upwards the flow of sex energy is also turned upwards, hence transforming the sexual energy into "spiritual energy".

Jalandhar Bandha

This bandha can be practised either along with internal pause (described in the process of normal breathing) or external pause by pressing the chin firmly against the chest and contracting the throat. This Bandh enhances the capacity of the pause for a longer period. This also helps in the union of prana with apana air and their entry into the sushmana nadi.

Maha Bandha

When all the three Bandhas *i.e.* Mool Bandh, Uddiyan Bandha and Jalandar Bandha are performed simultaneously at the same time, it is called "Maha Bandha". When the locks are opened or Bandhas are released, a particular sequence is followed. The Uddiyana Bandha is released first, followed by release of Jalandhar Bandh and Moola Bandha is released last of all.

Usually Bandhas are practised during the pause in breathing. Moola Bandha can be performed at any time during the process of breathing whereas Maha Bandha is performed at the time of external or internal pause. As a matter of fact any type of Bandha can be practised during "internal pause" of breathing.

Effects

Maha Bandha stabilises the vital energy (prana). Since prana controls the mind, the movement of the mind is determined by the movement of prana because the mind moves in the same direction in which the prana moves. Hence, stability of the mind is determined by the stability of the prana.

Techniques of Pranayam

Yogic Breathing: This forms the fundamental basis for

pranayam. *Yogic breath is a prolonged, deep, thin (noiseless) breath.*

Prolonged stands for greater duration (a normal person breathes 15 to18 times a minute, whereas a yogi breathes 10 to 12 times a minute and with practice 5 to 7 times a minute. In a prolonged breath, we take in more atmospheric air into our lungs. More air means more oxygen and more prana).

Deep breath means taking the atmospheric air to the deeper parts of the lungs particularly those air sacs which are situated at the bases or apex of the lungs so that there is uniform distribution of oxygen/ air in all parts of the lungs, irrespective of whether these parts are central, peripheral or situated at remote part of the lungs.

A *thin* breath is a uniform breath, which does not produce any sort of noise while passing through the respiratory passages. A thin breath is invariably a cool and uniform breath. Whereas a thick breath is a harsh breath, is a hot breath and is a haphazard breath.

The next stage of yogic breathing is its *regularity* and *rhythm*. A yogic breath is a controlled breath, which comes on at regular intervals and this regularity is developed with practice and should take a rhythmic form.

A yogi always tries to take yogic breaths irrespective of whether he is awake or asleep, whether he is walking, sitting or lying. He takes regular, deep, prolonged, noiseless breath all the time. A calm breath leads to calm mind. A calm mind can concentrate better, a concentrated mind can think better; a thinking mind can decide better, a decisive mind can act better.

Yogic breathing influences the Visuddha Chakra, which in turn makes the speech sweet and beautiful.

Gyan Mudra

Although this is not a pranayam, this is a posture, but, I believe it advisable to describe it in detail, as this posture needs to be performed for most of the pranayams.

Step 1: Sit in the lotus position or any other comfortable position with your spine erect and eyes shut.

Step 2: Flex the arms at the elbows; touch the tip of the index finger with the tip of the thumb (this means that the energy of the body shall not be expanded from the mini chakras present on the finger tips). Extend middle, ring and little finger (the mini chakras present on the finger tips help in imbibing the cosmic energy). Place the back of the wrists on the respective knees (see the photograph).

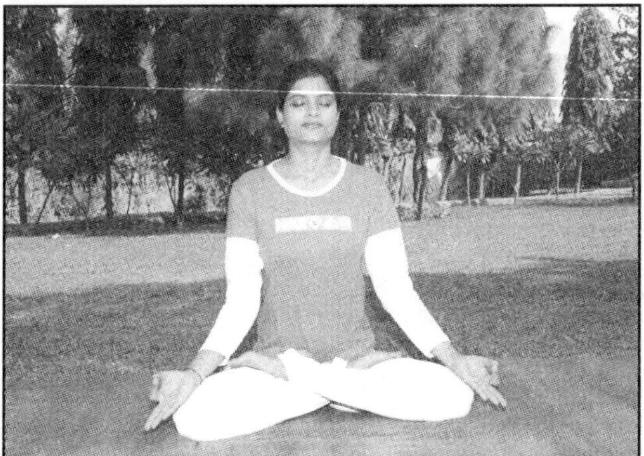

Gyan Mudra

Step 3: Take deep, prolonged, thin, yogic breaths.

Step 4: Concentrate (put your mind) on breathing.

Agni Sar Pranayam

As mentioned in the beginning most of the pranayams are performed in the lotus position or any other comfortable sitting position where the spine remains erect or upright. Agni Sar pranayam is performed in the following steps:

Step 1: Sit in the lotus position with an upright spine and hold both the knees with the respective hands firmly. The eyes are closed and the chin is brought slightly downwards towards the upper part of the chest.

Step 2: Take a deep breath through the nose, and fill both the lungs completely. This will make the abdominal muscles tight.

Step 3: Breathe out slowly and rhythmically so as to empty both the lungs making sure that your abdomen becomes completely soft. While breathing out apply Mool Bandha.

Step 4: Move the empty abdomen forwards and backwards a number of times till you feel like gasping for breath.

Step 5: Take prolonged, deep and rhythmical breaths.

This process may be repeated a number of times according to the body stamina.

Advantages

1. Agni Sar pranayam influences Manipur Chakra, which in turn helps in the process of digestion of various foods.

2. It helps in reducing the acid in the stomach, hence relieving chronic dyspepsia.
3. It also helps in reliving constipation and hardening the stools.

Brahmri Pranayam

Step 1: Sit in the lotus position, with your eyes closed and back in erect position. Place index and middle fingers on the eye, ring finger on the upper lip, little finger on the lower lip and thumb on the tragus of the ear, as shown in the photograph.

Step 2: Take a deep breath and fill the lungs with the air.

Step 3: Produce a humming sound while breathing out slowly through the nose.

Step 4: Repeat from step 2 onwards as many times as your body can cope.

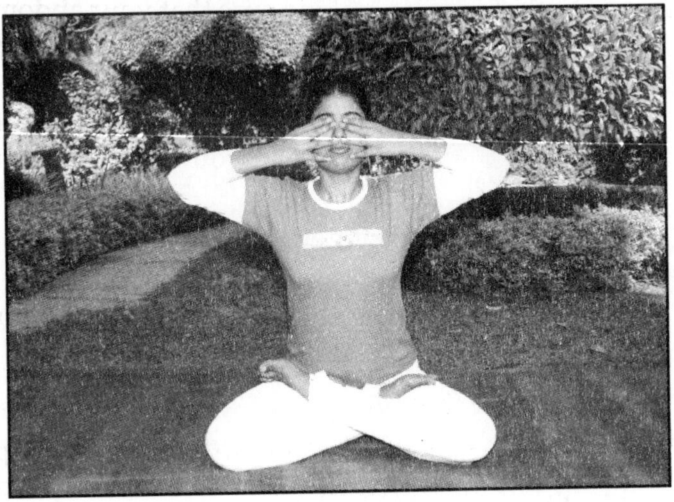

Brahmri Pranayam

Advantages

1. Brahmri Pranayam not only clears the nasal passages but it also clears the sinuses.
2. It vibrates the sinuses and the brain cells enhancing the memory.
3. This also opens the Eustachian tubes (tubes going from the back of the throat to the back of the ears, the air inside this tube keeps a balance between the inner air and the outer atmospheric air, hence enhancing the mechanism of hearing).
4. This is a very good pranayam for people who suffer from chronic sinusitis.

NADI SHODHAN PRANAYAM

Step 1: Sit in the lotus or any other comfortable position. Adopt "gyan mudra" on the left side by touching the tip of the left index finger with the tip of the thumb making a circle. The other three fingers are kept extended joined together. Keep the wrist on the bent knees as shown in the photograph.

Step 2: Bend the right arm at the elbow, keeping the elbow firmly with the body. Flex the index and middle finger on to the palm while thumb and ring finger remain extended the little finger is also extended but is kept away from the ring finger (see the photograph).

Step 3: Bring the thumb on to the right nostril and ring finger on to the left nostril.

Step 4: Block the right nostril with the thumb and inhale (breath in) through the left nostril, give a pause and slowly breathe out (exhale) from the right nostril while blocking the left nostril with the ring finger.

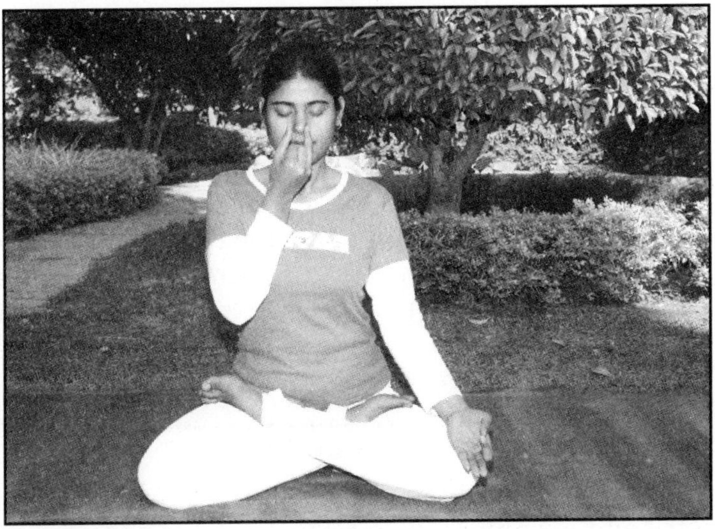

Nadi Shodhan (i)

In the beginning you should spend the same amount of time on inhaling, exhaling and pause e.g. if you spend 5 seconds on inhaling you should spend 5 seconds for pause and 5 seconds for exhaling (this is ratio of 1:1:1). Gradually you can increase this ratio to 1:2:2, 1:3:3 or 1:3:2 or may be 1:4:2 and so on. Exhaling should be complete so that every air sac of the lung is emptied.

This pranayam may be done by inhaling through the left nostril and exhaling through the right nostril. This is called *Candrika pranayam*

Or

It may be done by inhaling through the right nostril and exhaling through the left nostril. This is called *Surya pranayam.*

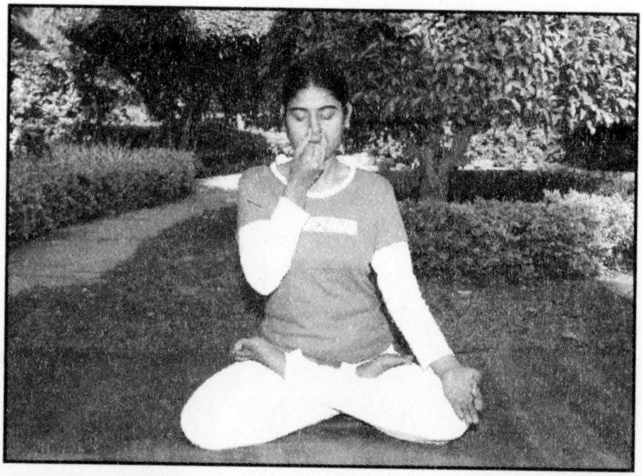

Nadi Shodhan (ii)

This may be done by inhaling through the left nostril and exhaling through the right nostril followed by inhaling through the right nostril and exhaling through the left nostril and this may be continued like this for as long as your body can cope. This is called *"Alome Vilome"*.There is no pause.

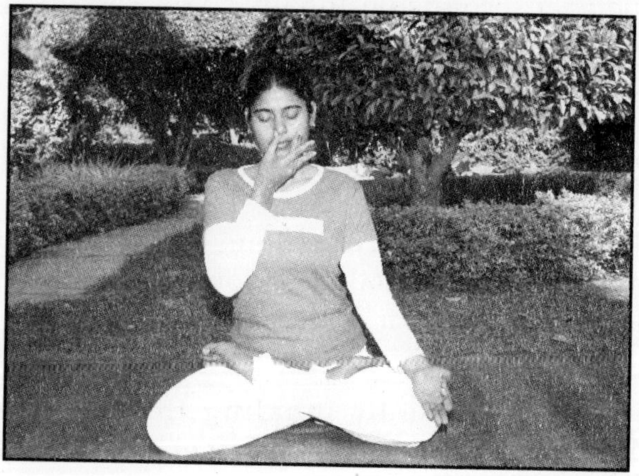

Nadi Shodhan (iii)

Effects

1. Nadi shodhan pranayam is supposed to energize all the six chakras (Chakra 1 to 6, see the chapter on Chakras).
2. It gets rid of all the old and wasted (utilized) energy from all seventy two thousand (72000) Nadis of the body and fills those Nadis with renewed and fresh energy.
3. In other words this pranayam energizes the whole body; hence this is called the king of pranayams.

Different stages of the Nadi shodhan pranayam are shown in the photograph.

Kapal Bhati Pranayam

Procedure

Step 1: Sit in the lotus or any other comfortable position, holding tightly your bent knees with your hands. Shut your eyes and keep your spine erect.

Step 2: Take a deep breath in (inhale) and fill both the lungs with the air.

Step 3: Release this air in small quantities with a jerk producing a noise through your nose. Every time you give a jerk, the diaphragm is pulled up and the abdomen goes in (a pit is produced in the stomach). Go on repeating the process till the air is let out from the lungs.

Step 4: Repeat steps 2 and 3 till you are gasping for breath.

Effects

1. This pranayam energizes Anahat Chakra as well as Vissudha Chakra.
2. This stimulates the diaphragm and is an excellent exercise for the diaphragm muscle.
3. This pranayam is excellent for people who suffer from hiccups.
4. This pranayam clears the respiratory passages and is an excellent exercise for the lungs.
5. This is a good pranayam for people who suffer from chronic condition of the lungs like Bronchial Asthma, Chronic Bronchitis and fibrosis of the lungs.

SHEETLI PRANAYAM

Sheetal means cool, hence this pranayam cools the body.

Procedure

Step 1: Sit in the lotus position or any other comfortable position adopting Gyan mudra, keeping your eyes closed.

Step 2: Pull your tongue out in between the closed lips. Fold the tongue from the sides and make a pipe of your tongue.

Step 3: Breath in through the pipe made out of the tongue producing a whistling noise, fill your lungs and mouth completely with the atmospheric air and hold your breath for a while.

Step 4: Breathe out completely through your nose.

Keep on repeating steps 3 and 4 as long as you can.

Effects

While you are sucking the air in through the pipe, cool energy runs throughout your body, which gives calming effects to the nerves and the mind.

This is an excellent pranayam for cooling the heat of the summer or when the outside atmospheric temperature is high.

Sheetkari Pranayam

This also cools the body and is a good procedure to be performed when the atmospheric temperature is high.

Procedure

Step 1: Clinch your teeth, while front part of the tongue remains stuck to the hard palate.

Step 2: Breath in (inhale) through the clinched teeth and feel the cooling effect of the atmospheric air as it passes in between your teeth. Fill your lung as much as you can and hold your breath for a while.

Step 3: Breathe out completely through the nose.

Repeat steps 2 and 3 a few times or as long as you can.

Effects

This pranayam not only has a cooling effect on your teeth and mouth but it has a cooling effect on all the energy running in your nadis.

Sheetli and Sheet Kari are usually performed one after the other for their cooling effect to the body, mind and nerves.

Ujjayi Pranayam

Ujjayi means upward or superior, which may also be interpreted as "expended". In this pranayam, the lungs are fully expanded and chest is puffed out, keeping the abdomen absolutely still.

Procedure

Step 1: Sit in padamasana or any other comfortable position. Adopt the Gyan mudra position and close the eyes.

Step 2: Breathe out (exhale) completely.

Step 3: Inhale slowly but steadily through both the nostrils and try to feel the incoming air on the roof of the palate. You are likely to hear a low velocity sound (Ujjayi).

Step 4: Fill both the lungs completely bringing the chest out but making sure that the abdomen does not become prominent.

Step 5: Pull the entire abdomen backwards towards the spine and hold the breath till you feel choked.

Step 6: Breathe out (exhale) slowly, deeply and empty the lungs completely. While exhaling again feel the passage of air against your palate and appreciate the hustling noise of air.

Step 7: Wait for a few seconds and repeat the process from step 3 to step 6.

The process may be repeated as many times as your body can tolerate

Effects

(1) Ujjayi pranayam is helpful in removing the phlegm from the lungs; it tones the entire respiratory system.

(2) It has a soothing effect on the nerves.

(3) This is a useful pranayam for people suffering

from high blood pressure and coronary heart disease.

Bhasrika Pranayam

This is an excellent pranayam for strengthening the lungs. It is performed in the following steps:

Step 1: Exhale and empty your lungs completely.

Step 2: Take sharp and shallow breaths and keep on increasing their crescendo, reach a peak and bring the crescendo back. Repeat this as many times as you can.

Step 3: Fill your lungs with a deep prolonged breath and hold your breath.

Step 4: Slowly breathe out and completely empty your lungs.

Step 5: Breathe normally.

Advantages

(1) It helps in clearing the nasal passages.

(2) It strengthens the lungs by increasing the elasticity of the lungs.

(3) It exercises the intercostal muscles as well as the ribs, hence it makes the rib cage stronger.

(4) It increases the vital capacity of the lungs.

Many other techniques of pranayam have been described for which I recommended a reference book on pranayams.

Yoga Energy System

4

YOGA ENERGY SYSTEM

Human energy is spread over four phases:

(1) Spiritual

(2) Mental

(3) Emotional

(4) Physical

Physical ⟶ Emotional ⟶ Mental ⟶ Spiritual

A block anywhere in this pathway can jeopardise the energy system. Plato said: "soul is a unity of forces liable to fly apart."

A sustained mental and emotional development is required to open spiritual pathway. In modern civilisation Intellect (mind) rules over the Spirit and Emotions, hence making the mental body supreme.

Intellectuals are less emotional and ignore the physical body. It is difficult to develop spirituality with a highly developed intellect.

Intellect + emotion = spiritual development.

The energy body which immediately surrounds the physical body is called the "etheric body".

Energy to the physical body comes from outside as well as from the food we eat. Outside energy is supplied by the "etheric body", which is situated outside the physical body. It conforms to the shape and size of the physical body and is also called the bio-plasmic body or Aura.

This bio-plasmic body has a definite and well laid out system, which acts as a receiving and distributing station of energy for the physical body, for performance of vital functions.

The bio-plasmic body or etheric body gets energy from cosmos, sun and various other sources such as sound and vibrations etc. This energy is received by manholes called Chakras, which are circular whirlpools of energy distributed all over the body. There are Mini Chakras and Minor Chakras on the hands and the feet.

This refined form of energy is circulated throughout the etheric body in channels, which are as thin as hair and are called nadis. There are 72000 – 125000 nadis spread all over the etheric body which are classified into large, medium and small nadis depending upon their length and diameter. All these nadis pass through or around, criss-cross, overlap, join each other, at the level of the navel (belly button) of the physical body. It shows aggregation and intensity of the energy at this particular place.

The physical body also derives energy from food, which is a comparatively crude form of energy. This combined with the energy derived from the bio-plasmic body helps in the performance of various functions of different parts/ organs/ systems of the physical body.

The energy system of the bio-plasmic body is very well developed along the spinal column (backbone), where the energy runs from bottom to top and vice versa passing through the energy wells, which act as relay stations of the energy. These relay stations are called

"Major Chakras", and are six (6) in number. These Chakras are situated in the energy body along the spinal column and are called:

Mooladhara Chakra
Svadishthana Chakra
Manipura Chakra
Anahata Chakra
Vissudha Chakra and
Ajna Chakra.

The main nadi, which runs through the centre of these Chakras, is called "Sushmana Nadi". Two other main nadis called 'Ida' and 'Pingla' run along the left and the right side of the Chakras respectively from below upwards criss-crossing and embracing the Chakras, reaching the Ajna Chakra where the 'Ida' is connected to the outside atmosphere through the left nostril and the 'Pingla' is connected to the outside air through the right nostril.

A brief description of these Chakras and three main nadis is given below. For a detailed concept of the energy system of the body the reader should refer to the book, *Vital Energy* by the same author.

Mooladhara Chakra

This is situated at the tail end of the spine (backbone) and represents the element earth. This Chakra influences the adrenal glands for the release of their hormones (corticosteroids). This Chakra also influences stomach, intestines, the blood system, bones, muscles and immune system of the body.

The main function of this Chakra is to keep the body in harmony with nature, rooting the body, giving it security and desire for survival and expansion.

Svadishthana Chakra

This Chakra is situated in the pelvic region behind the genitalia and represents the element water, which means different excretions and secretions, which take place around that area. Hence, it influences the testes in the male, which produce semen and male hormone (testosterone) and ovaries in females, which produce ovum and estrogens (female hormone). This Chakra also influences the kidneys, urinary bladder, reproductive organs, and it helps in expelling the waste products from the body. It also helps in the extension of the progeny through the process of love-making.

This Chakra acts as a centre for sexual energy, source of pure emotions and regulator of relationships.

Manipura Chakra

This is situated at the level of the navel (belly button) and represents the element fire. Besides influencing the liver and pancreas it also influences adrenal glands. Pancreatic secretions, production and storage of bile, movement of the small intestines are all influenced through the sympathetic nervous system by this chakra.

This Chakra gives autonomy to an individual, who develops "self-esteem" and tolerance. "Self-esteem" brings in the power and the ego identity.

Anahat Chakra

This Chakra is located in the chest near the heart and represents the element air. Basically, this Chakra influences the thymus gland, which is situated at the upper part of the sternum (central chest bone). It also influences the heart, lungs, circulation of the blood and vagus nerves. Vagus nerves supply the heart as well as the stomach. So this Chakra indirectly influences the stomach. When a person becomes emotional and the vagus nerves are stimulated, it not only affects the heart but also the person feels a funny sensation in the stomach.

The main function of this Chakra is to impart a feeling of love to a person. It also comes into play in the development of relationships, intimacy and devotion. Hence this Chakra has got everything to do with the emotions and feelings.

Vissudha Chakra

Located in the neck at the level of the throat, the Vissudha Chakra is blue in colour. It represents the element sound, which requires air for its production. This Chakra influences the thyroid and parathyroid glands which are situated almost in the middle of the neck. This Chakra also influences the larynx (sound box), respiratory system and vagus nerves (the function of the vagus nerves has already been described).

This Chakra is related to the process of phonation, communication and expression of ideas and thoughts which mean inner reflection of an individual.

Ajna Chakra

This is located on the forehead between the two eyebrows and represents the element 'Ether'. The Ajna Chakra influences the pineal gland, pituitary gland and hypothalamus, which are all situated inside the brain. It indirectly influences the left eye and the nose.

This Chakra connects the individual to the rest of creation through the process of intuition, visualisation, imagination and dreaming. This Chakra is also involved with pattern recognition.

Sahasrara Chakra

Although Sahasrara Chakra is not a part of the Chakra system along the spine (backbone), but this is most important Chakra situated above the head, which connects the person with the Cosmos. This Chakra influences the pineal gland, thalamus and hypothalamus, which are all parts of the brain. In other words it influences the functions of the higher brain as well as the right eye.

This Chakra makes a person aware of universal identity, spirituality and divinity. Through this Chakra human vital energy is connected with the cosmic energy.

A brief description of the three main nadis is given below:

Sushmana Nadi

This nadi connects the Mooladhara Chakra with the Sahasrara Chakra, passing through the centre of the other five Chakras *i.e.* Svadishthana, Manipura, Anahata, Vissudha and Ajna Chakras. This is supposed to be the main nadi supplying energy to all the Chakras and also acting as a channel of communication between the Chakras.

Kundalini Shakti, which lies dormant in the Mooladhara Chakra, rises up and traverses the Sushmana Nadi. This nadi facilitates the process of meditation and spirituality.

Ida Nadi

This also begins from Mooladhara Chakra, is smaller in diameter than the Sushmana nadi and runs along the left side of the spinal column. While ascending it crosses over to the other side near a Chakra embracing that Chakra, after reaching the Ajna Chakra, it descends downwards along the left nostril and establishes its connection with the outside atmosphere. It is said to carry cool energy.

Pingla Nadi

This also begins from the Mooladhara Chakra, runs upwards along the right side of the spinal column. It is slightly bigger in diameter than the Ida Nadi. It criss-crosses on to the other side near the Chakra, hence embracing the Chakra partially, after having reached Ajna Chakra it descends along the right nostril to establish its communication with the outside atmosphere. It is supposed to carry hot energy.

It is thought that people who take the path of spirituality via Pingla nadi go through the path of knowledge, whereas people who follow the path of spirituality through Ida nadi go by the path of devotion.

The energy supplied to the body by food has been described in the section on "Yoga and Diet."

Yoga and Diet

5

Yoga and Diet

Food is the main energy provider for the human body. Energy is not only needed for growth, development and other activities of life, but also for the performance of the vital activities of the body such as respiration, beating of the heart, circulation of the blood and digestion of the food. The ability of human beings to meet their nutritional needs and maintain good health depends upon the type and the quality of the food they eat.

Dietary habits of populations in different regions of the world have been determined mainly by the availability of the foods locally as well as by local practices. Humans have evolved their eating habits by a process of trial and error. Satisfaction of hunger is usually the primary criterion but it is not a safe guide for selection of proper foods. For leading a healthy and active life the diet should be based on sound "nutritional principles".

Thousands of years ago, our ancestors based their recommendations regarding a balanced diet, keeping in view the foods available at that time. Since then there has been a great revolution not only in the variety of foods but also in our eating habits. With industrialisation and advancement in technology different communities now do not depend on the foods available locally. Foods are imported from all over the world to satisfy the taste buds.

Before I embark upon explanation of the diets recommended to lead a life of a yogi, I would like to make the reader wiser regarding a "balanced diet" because this has become the burning issue of the day. In olden days because of the scarcity of the food, people used to die of malnutrition, nowadays food is available in abundance and those people who can afford it die of over eating (obesity) and its effects.

It is essential for every person to have some basic knowledge about the food we eat, and the purpose it serves. Keeping this in mind I wish to explain in the following pages the basic nutrients required by each individual for the sustenance of the body. These nutrients include proteins, fats, carbohydrates, vitamins and minerals.

Depending upon the relative compositions of these nutrients, food is classified as:

Protein rich food

Carbohydrates rich food and

Fat rich food.

There are lots of foods which only provide a single nutrient *e.g.* sugars are only a source of carbohydrates, while oil and ghee are only providers of fat. Lots of other foods provide multiple nutrients, such as milk provides proteins, carbohydrates as well as fat. Similarly wheat provides proteins, carbohydrates and even fat to an extent. The main function of proteins, besides providing energy to the body, is to provide amino acids for building body proteins. Fats, besides being a concentrated source of energy also provide essential fatty acids, which have a vitamin like function in body. Vegetables and fruits (foods from plant origin) also contain fiber, which is indigestible but has a useful function in the process of digestion and formation of stools.

Vitamins and minerals do not supply energy to the body as such but play a very important role in regulation of metabolic activity of the body by performing certain chemical reactions in the body. Minerals also play an important role for the formation of body structures like bones and muscles.

Human bodies need the entire above-mentioned nutrients in different amounts for their growth, so the human diet must be a well balanced diet providing all these nutrients in proper proportions. I shall make an effort to describe the different nutrients in more detail for the benefit of the reader, because food and sex play the most important role in the lives of human beings. I shall deal with sex in the subsequent chapter. At present we shall confine ourselves to food.

Proteins

Proteins are important constituents of the cells as well as tissues of the body. The whole body is made up of billions of cells and so many different varieties of tissues, so you can imagine the importance of proteins in tissue building including blood formation. Proteins provide the body with the building material and make good the loss that occurs due to wear and tear. Hence proteins are vital to the living process because they carry out a wide range of functions essential for the sustenance of life.

Proteins which we take in our diet are broken down into amino acids, which in turn are synthesised by the body into proteins to be replaced into the tissues. Those amino acids, which are not used in protein synthesis, are broken down to provide energy to the body.

Amino acids work as body building blocks; they protect the cells, relieve pain, generate ecstasy and act as food for fulfillment of sexual activities. In short they are guardians of health. The whole process of well being of the body depends upon amino acids. They can protect us by shielding us from radiation, pollution and can slow down the aging process. Free form amino acids can also help against allergies and auto immune diseases.

One gram of protein gives rise to 4.2 kcal of energy. (The energy unit of the body is expressed in Kcal; this shall be described under a separate heading so as to make the reader understand what it means and how it is calculated.) Proteins in the diet are most economically used for the formation of body proteins.

Sources of proteins

All foods except sugars and oils contain proteins in varying degrees. Foods which contain high amounts of protein are classified as protein rich foods and examples of such foods are meat, fish and eggs from animal source, pulses, oil seeds and nuts from vegetable source. Milk is an important source of protein but can be derived from both animal as well as vegetable sources.

Soya bean is the richest source containing over 40% of protein.

Cereals are a moderate source of protein; they contain 10% of protein.

Rice contains 7% proteins but these are better quality proteins as compared to wheat and other cereals.

Cereals are consumed in large quantities everyday, hence they contribute a considerate amount of protein to the daily intake.

Leafy vegetables, fruits, roots and tubers are poor sources of protein because they contain less than 2% of protein.

Defatted oil seeds are the richest sources of proteins, as they contain 50 to 60 % of proteins. Defatted oil seeds are available for human consumption these days whereas in the past these have been usually used for feeding animals and chickens.

Nutritional value of protein

Proteins present in different foods vary in their nutritional quality because of the differences in the amino acid composition. Amino acids are the building blocks of proteins, and proteins are broken into different amino acids. There are 19 amino acids in proteins, which have been described so far. Out of these, 9 of them are designated as "essential amino acids". Essential amino acids cannot be synthesised in the body. Those amino acids which can be synthesised in the body are called non-essential amino acids because they can be formed in the body by interconversion of other essential amino acids.

The best quality protein is the one which provides essential amino acids very close to the pattern of the tissue proteins. Only two proteins satisfy these criteria and are classified as high quality proteins, these are egg proteins and human milk proteins. Egg proteins serve as reference proteins for defining the quality of other proteins.

Proteins of animal foods like milk, meat, fish etc. generally compare well with egg protein in their essential amino acid composition and are categorised as high-class proteins and these proteins are easily digested.

Plant proteins on the other hand are lower class proteins. In comparison to egg proteins, cereal proteins are poor in the amino acid 'lysine', on the other hand, pulses and oil seed proteins are rich in lysine but are poor in sulphur containing amino acids. Such proteins individually are incomplete proteins. However this insufficiency of a particular amino acid can be overcome by combining with other vegetable foods which are rich in that particular amino acid, hence a cereal taken along with pulses can overcome this deficiency.

Another factor in assessing the value of proteins in a foodstuff is its digestibility. Proteins of uncooked vegetable foods particularly pulses are less easily digested than those of animal foods. Hence cooking improves the digestibility of proteins in several foods.

From the above discussion it becomes very clear that the nutritional value of food depends upon its essential amino acid make-up and its digestibility. The protein value of cereal can be improved by addition of leafy vegetables.

Body requirements of proteins

Proteins are required for repair of wear and tear of tissues in adults, for growth in children, for fetal development in pregnancy and during lactation.

Requirement for the last three categories is more than the requirement of the first category. The better the quality of the protein, the lower the requirement and vice versa. The adult requirement of first class protein is from 0.7 gm per kg of body weight, while requirement of mixed vegetable protein is 1 gm per kg of body weight. Children require about 1.2 gm per kg of body weight of superior quality proteins and the same requirement holds true during pregnancy and lactation.

Protein content of the whole diet should be enough to contribute around 10% of the total caloric requirements of the body. This requirement is increased to about 15% in growing children, pregnant mothers and lactating women.

Eggs besides providing superior quality protein are also rich in vitamin B12, which is absent in the vegetarian diet. Skimmed milk and buttermilk also serve as good sources of superior quality proteins.

Fats

Fat is an important part of the diet because in the time of need it supplies a concentrated form of energy, which is more than twice the energy provided by the same amount of carbohydrates or proteins.

Fat gives shape to the body.

Fat makes food palatable.

Fat delays the emptying of the stomach, which means that a person does not feel hungry for a long time after eating a fatty meal.

Fat is an important source for fat-soluble vitamins particularly vitamin A.

Fat, particularly derived from vegetable sources, provides essential fatty acids, which have vitamin-like functions in the body.

Dietary fat can be of two forms:

(1) Visible fat is derived from animal sources like

butter, ghee, milk etc, it can also be derived from vegetable sources like groundnut, mustard, coconut, sunflower and various other vegetable oils.

Hydrogenated vegetable oils are solid fat known as vanaspathi which is popular in India.

These visible fats are in the form of triglycerides of fatty acids, which may be saturated as well as unsaturated.

Saturated fatty acids are predominantly found in animal fats whereas unsaturated fatty acids dominate in vegetable oils.

Animal fats like ghee and butter also contain Vitamins A and D, which are not present in vegetable oils, but can be added.

(2) Invisible fat—Some amount of fat which is not apparently visible is present in various other foods like cereals, pulses, egg, meat, etc. This invisible fat is believed to contribute significantly to the total body fat. It is a wrong notion that nations, which eat mainly cereals and pulses, do not become overweight.

A cereal-pulse based diet not containing any visible fat but can provide more than 50% of the requirement of the essential fatty acids in an individual.

In modern times when food is eaten for the sake of pleasure and to satisfy the palate and not to satisfy hunger, the excessive intake of fat in the diet increases the level of cholesterol in the blood, which is deposited in the arteries and may block the smaller arteries. When the coronary arteries supplying the heart get blocked, it may lead to a heart attack.

It has been observed that if more than 80 gms of saturated fats are eaten per day, it leads to an increase in the blood cholesterol. Keeping in mind the nutritional significance of unsaturated fatty acids found in vegetable oils, these not only act as a source of essential fatty acids required by the body but also help in the control of blood cholesterol.

Essential fatty acids play an important role in several metabolic reactions in the body and their deficiency may lead to certain medical problems particularly roughening of the skin.

On one hand a high proportion of saturated fats (LDL) in butter, ghee and hydrogenated oils have shown to cause considerable elevation of blood cholesterol, on the other hand unsaturated (HDL) fatty acids present in vegetable oils particularly groundnut oil, olive oil, sunflower oil, rice bran oil, have been shown to prevent the increase in blood cholesterol. Hence, these oils are considered to be friendly for the human body.

In addition to the quantity and quality, the mode of consumption of fat also appears to influence the blood cholesterol levels. The consumption of a small quantity of fat several times a day has been shown to cause less elevation of blood cholesterol as compared to consumption of fat in larger quantities at one time.

Body requirements of fats

In deciding the desirable level of fat in the diet the following facts have to be considered:

(1) The minimum amount of fat required, meeting the essential fatty acid requirements of the body.

(2) The amount of fat needed to promote

absorption of fat-soluble vitamins *i.e.* Vitamin A, D, E and K.

(3) The amount of fat providing sufficient palatability to the food.

(4) The undesirable effects of excessive intake of fat.

The essential fatty acid requirement of a normal human body is 3-6 per cent of the total energy intake. This requirement is higher in growing children, during pregnancy and lactation. To obtain this level, the amount of visible fat taken in the diet should be between 15-25 gms per day preferably taken in the form of vegetable oils particularly groundnut oil. Even a predominantly cereal based diet would provide 15 gms fat, which is equal to 50% of the essential fatty acid requirement. One should endeavor not to exceed 30% of the total caloric intake in the form of fat.

1 gm of fat = 9Kcal

Carbohydrates

Carbohydrates are purely energy generating substances, which include starch, glucose and various other sugars like milk sugar, cane sugar, etc. Starch is a complex carbohydrate whereas sugars are simpler carbohydrates. Starch and other sugars need to be converted into glucose by the body for the production of energy. Wheat, which is eaten all over the world contains starch as its main ingredient.

There is no difference in starch from different sources. Lots of foods contain starch as well as an indigestible carbohydrate in the form of "dietary fiber". The fiber is not digested, hence it does not provide any energy but contributes to the bulk of stools allowing the individual not to be constipated. Some of the dietary fibers like gums and mucilage in our diet have been shown to lower blood cholesterol and blood sugar. Cereals are comparatively rich in fiber. People who perform physical labour should be given carbohydrate rich food in sufficient quantity to meet their energy demands.

Body requirements of carbohydrates

About 50 to 60% of the energy for the body is derived from carbohydrates.

1 gm of carbohydrate = about 4Kcal of energy.

The daily requirement of carbohydrate for an adult male is between 300-350 gms.

Daily diet of an adult should contain at least 40 gms of dietary fiber.

VITAMINS

Vitamins are present in small amounts in many foods.

Vitamins are required for carrying out many vital functions of the body.

Vitamins are involved in the utilization of other major nutrients like carbohydrates, fat and proteins.

Vitamins are needed in small amounts but are essential for the health and well being of the body.

Vitamins act as catalytic agents in so many chemical reactions inside the body.

Vitamins are classified into two groups:

(1) *Fat-soluble vitamins:* these vitamins dissolve in the fat, hence can be stored in the body fat and may prove injurious to health if taken in large quantities. Fat-soluble vitamins are Vitamins A, D, E and K.

(2) *Water-soluble vitamins:* these vitamins being soluble in water are readily excreted, hence are not stored in the body, so they do not have any toxic effects on the body. Main water-soluble vitamins are vitamin B complex and vitamin C.

Vitamin A

This is also called 'Retinol'. The word 'retinol' is derived from retina, which is a curtain at the back of the eye, because this vitamin is an ingredient of a fluid called "visual purple", which is produced by the retina and helps people in seeing clearly in the dark. Deficiency of this vitamin causes "night blindness".

Vitamin A can also be derived from carotene present in carrots as their yellow pigment. Other sources of Vitamin A are butter, ghee, milk, yogurt, egg yolk and liver particularly liver oils of certain fishes like cod, halibut and shark. Other sources of carotene are green leafy vegetables mangoes, papaya, tomatoes, pumpkins and red palm oil.

Vitamin A also maintains the integrity of the epithelial tissues. Its deficiency may affect the epithelium of the eyes producing dry eyes. The daily requirement of Vitamin A for an adult is about 2500 international units. Intake of a large amount of vitamin A for prolonged periods may lead to toxic symptoms, which include irritability, headache, nausea and vomiting.

Vitamin D

Vitamin D plays an important part in absorption of calcium from the intestines and in its deposition in the bones; hence this is an essential vitamin for the growth of bones and for calcium metabolism.

Lack of Vitamin D in the diet, leads to rickets (bowed legs) in children and osteomalacia (brittle bones) in adults. Osteomalacia manifests as pain in the bones, is more common in women, and usually starts during pregnancy. Ultimately the bones of the victim become brittle and start bending, making the victim unable to stand and develop a pelvic tilt, that is why it is recommended that women should drink large quantities of milk during pregnancy which is a source of calcium as well as Vitamin D.

Other sources of Vitamin D are butter and ghee, but the most important source of Vitamin D, which is free for all, is sunlight. Vitamin D is formed in the skin by the action of ultra violet rays present in the sunlight.

Body requirement of Vitamin D

Vitamin D requirement of a developing child is between 200 to 400 international units and all of this may be obtained from the sunlight in tropical countries. 1 gm of pure Vitamin D equals 40 million international units.

Excessive amount of Vitamin D in the body can lead to similar toxic symptoms produced by excessive intake of Vitamin A, which include irritability, nausea, vomiting and constipation.

Vitamin K

This is another fat-soluble vitamin and is widely distributed in the plant and animal kingdom. It helps in the process of coagulation (clotting) of blood.

Vitamin E

Like Vitamin K, Vitamin E is also fat-soluble and is found in various plants and foods of animal origin.

It is present in high concentrations in vegetable oils and cereals. Vitamin E possesses anti-oxidant properties. There is a wrong belief that Vitamin E acts as a sex tonic, which has not been proved by any authentic study. Vitamin E is said to revitalize the skin. Daily requirement of Vitamin E in humans is not known with certainty.

Vitamin B

B vitamins have various components from vitamin B1 to B12. From the health point of view B1 (Thiamine), B2 (Riboflavin), Nicotinic acid, pyridoxine (B6), Folic acid and vitamin B12 are important.

Thiamine is an anti-neuritis vitamin and its deficiency leads to Polly neuritis. The richest source of thiamine is yeast, outer layer of rice, wheat, millets, pulses and nuts particularly groundnuts.

Daily thiamine requirement ranges between 0.5 to 2 mgm.

Riboflavin is essential for several oxidation processes inside the cell and is concerned with energy production and protein metabolism.

Sore tongue and cracking at the angles of the mouth are produced due to lack of riboflavin. Eczema of the scrotum has also been reported due to lack of this vitamin in the diet. Good sources of riboflavin are milk, milk products, eggs, liver, leafy vegetables, wheat, pulses and millets. Daily dietary requirement of this vitamin ranges from 0.7 to 2.2 mgm depending upon the age.

Nicotinic Acid: This vitamin takes part in different oxidative reactions in the body and is concerned with metabolism of almost all the nutrients including carbohydrates, fats and proteins.

Lack of this vitamin in the diet leads to a disease called 'pellagra', which is characterised by sore tongue, pigmented skin and diarrhea. Pellagra is more common in the maize eating population because maize is a poor source of nicotinic acid. Whole cereals, pulses, nuts particularly groundnut and meat are good sources of nicotinic acid.

Daily requirement of nicotinic acid is between 0.6 to 2.5 mgm depending upon the age.

Pyridoxine: This is also called vitamin B6, which helps in metabolism of proteins and fat. Deficiency of this vitamin has not been defined clearly, it has been reported to cause convulsions in children and cracking of the corners of the lips in adults. It is thought that the daily intake of vitamin B6 between 0.6 to 2.5 mgm would meet the requirements of different age groups. Meat, liver, vegetables and whole cereal grains are good sources of vitamin B6.

Folic acid: This is one of the two vitamins of the B series to be associated with a certain type of anemia, because this is required for maturation of the red blood cells. The daily requirement of folic acid is between 50 to 100 micro grams. However this requirement is increased during pregnancy to 150-300 micro grams. Folic acid is found in animal as well as plant foods such as green vegetables, liver, pulses, etc.

Vitamin B12: Like folic acid B12 is also involved in the maturation of red blood cells and deficiency of B12 leads to a form of anemia. Vitamin B12 is also required for proper functioning of the central nervous system and for metabolism of folic acid. The human daily requirement of this vitamin is about 1micro gram. Vitamin B12 is synthesized by bacteria from animal foods; hence its deficiency is more common in vegetarians. Vitamin B12 is found in traces in lots of vegetables.

Vitamin C (ascorbic acid): This vitamin is an essential nutrient for human beings because they lack the capacity to synthesis ascorbic acid in the body. Ascorbic acid is a strong reducing agent and is involved in the synthesis of collagen tissue, bone, calcification of teeth and many more reactions in the body. Deficiency of Vitamin C causes Scurvy, which means weak bleeding gums; it also causes defective bone growth. Vitamin C helps in the absorption of iron. It is widely found in plant foods particularly fresh citrus fruits, like oranges, lemons, grapes etc. The richest and cheapest source of Vitamin C is Amla. A single amla supplies all the daily needs of Vitamin C. Vitamin C is destroyed in dry and stale vegetables. So it is advisable to eat raw fresh vegetables for the requirements of Vitamin C. Dry grains or pulses do not contain any Vitamin C but when dry pulses or beans are allowed to germinate Vitamin C is formed during the process of germination. Heating or drying the fresh vegetables usually destroys most of the Vitamin C.

Minerals and Metals

A large number of minerals and metals are present in the body. Some of them form part of the different tissues whereas others act as catalytic agents in many body reactions. For example, bones are made up mainly of calcium, magnesium and phosphorus; iron forms a content of the blood, minerals like zinc, copper, manganese and magnesium take part in a lot of enzyme systems of the body; iodine is excreted in an hormone called thyroxin; sodium and potassium form important parts of intra and extra cellular fluids (body fluids); bicarbonate and carbonates are helpful in keeping the acid base equilibrium of the body.

With this much basic knowledge of the diet we now proceed to the energy system.

ENERGY FOR THE BODY

As mentioned earlier, energy in the body is required for:

(1) Rest
(2) Activity
(3) Growth

Rest

It is understood that the body expends a certain amount of energy for essential functions like respiration, heartbeat, blood circulation, digestion, absorption, excretion and maintenance of body temperature.

The amount of energy expended when the body is at complete rest both physically as well as mentally is called "resting metabolism" or "basal metabolism". This is influenced by age, sex, height, weight and state of nutrition of the individual.

Basal metabolism for a given age and sex is taken as a starting point for calculating the total energy requirement of an individual body.

Activity

Activity means body activity of different individuals which includes manual work (which may be light or heavy), sitting, walking, and running, dressing and performing various functions required by the profession of an individual. The energy required for this activity is about one and a half times the basal energy.

Growth

Extra energy is required for growth of the body, hence more energy is required for growing children.

The three main components which provide body energy are carbohydrates, which should provide roughly 50 - 60% of the total body requirement of the energy.

Proteins should provide 10 to 15% of the total body energy requirements.

It is desirable that energy provided by fat should not exceed 30% of the total energy requirement of the body.

Unit of energy

The energy provided by different constituents of food has been measured in terms of calories.

Calorie being such a small unit the energy measurement of different foods is done in kilocalorie (Kcal), which is 1000 times the physical caloric unit.

Definition of Kilocalorie (Kcal)

The amount of heat required to raise the temperature of one kilogram of water by one degree centigrade (from 14.5C to 15.5C), is equal to 1kilocalorie.

A new energy unit has been introduced recently by the International Union of Nutritional Sciences and is called the Joule. Joule is defined as the energy required to move 1 kilogram mass 1 meter by 1 newton (1 newton is the force needed to accelerate one kilogram by one meter per second square, 1 kg by 1 m per se2).

Hence one calorie = 4.184 Joule or 1 kilo calorie= 4.184 kilo Joule

As mentioned earlier the total energy requirement of an individual is made up of two components:

(1) Basal energy requirement

(2) Energy required for the physical activity of the individual.

The energy consumption of an average male doing a sedentary job is 2400 Kcal/day (this is taken as 1 unit of the coefficient).

An adult male doing moderately heavy work requires about 2800 Kcal/day.

An adult male doing heavy work requires about 3600 Kcal/day.

An adult female doing a sedentary job requires about 2000 Kcalories.

An adult female doing moderately heavy work requires 2200 Kcalories.

An adult female doing a heavy job requires 280 Kcalories.

Requirements for growing children may vary from 1000 Kcalories to 2000 Kcalories depending upon their age. This requirement is increased in women during pregnancy and lactation.

For the benefit of the reader, the caloric values of commonly consumed foods are given in the subsequent pages.

Kilocaloric value of commonly consumed foods

All the values are per 100 gms of edible portion

Cereal grains and products	
Bajra (Bujri seeds)	361
Barley	336
Italian millet	331
Jowar	349
Maize, dry	342
Maize, tender	125
Rice, raw hand pounded	346
Rice, raw milled	345
Rice, puffed	325
Wheat, whole	346
Wheat, flour (whole)	341
Wheat, flour (refined)	348
Wheat, bread (brown)	244
Wheat, bread (white)	245
Pulses & Legumes	
Bengal gram, whole	360
Black gram, dhal	347
Lentil	343
Peas green	93
Peas dry	315
Rajmah (Red beans)	346
Soya beans	432
Leafy Vegetables	
Amaranth (tender)	45
Betel leaves	44
Brussels sprouts	52
Cabbage	27
Celery leaves	37

Celery stalk	18
Coriander leaves	44
Curry leaves	108
Garden Cress	67
Lettuce	21
Mint	48
Mustard Leaves	34
Parsley	87
Spinach	26
Roots & Tubers	
Arrow root flour	334
Beet root	43
Carrot	48
Onion (big)	50
Onion (small)	59
Parsnip	111
Potato	97
Radish, pink	32
Radish, white	17
Sweet potato	120
Turnip	29
Vegetables	
Runner beans	158
Bottle gourd	12
Brinjal (aubergenes) or Egg plant	24
Broad beans	48
Cauliflower	30
Cluster beans	16
Cucumber	13

French beans	26
Ladies finger	35
Leeks	77
Lotus stems (dry)	234
Mango (green)	44
Pumpkin fruit	25
Tinda	21
Tomatoes	23
Water chestnut	115
Nuts & Oil Seeds	
Almonds	655
Cashew nut	596
Chilgoza	615
Coconut (dry)	662
Coconut (fresh)	444
Coconut tender	41
Coconut milk	430
Coconut water	24
Groundnut	567
Groundnut roasted	570
Linseed seeds	530
Pistachio nut	626
Sunflower seed	620
Walnut	687
Spices & Condiments	
Asafetida	297
Cardamom	229
Chilies dry	246
Chilies green	29

Cloves dry	286
Coriander whole	286
Cumin seeds	356
Garlic dry	145
Ginger fresh	67
Lime peel	129
Mango power	337
Nutmeg fruit	472
Nutmeg rind	52
Black pepper (dry)	304
Pepper green	98
Pippali	310
Turmeric	349
Fruits	
Amla	58
Apple	59
Apricot fresh	53
Avocado	215
Banana	116
Gooseberry	53
Cherries	64
Currants black	316
Dates, dried	317
Dates, fresh	144
Figs	37
Grapes, black	58
Grapes, green	71
Grape fruit	45
Guava	51

Lemon	57
Litchi	61
Lime	59
Mango	74
Melon	60
Water melon	16
Orange	48
Orange juice	9
Papaya, ripe	32
Passion fruit	54
Peaches	50
Pears	52
Pineapple	46
Plum	52
Pomegranate	65
Prunes	56
Raisins	308
Raspberry	56
Strawberry	44
Sea Food	
Bombay duck, dried	293
Cat fish	86
Chingri, (small dried)	292
Crab, small	169
Herring	119
Lobster	90
Mackerel	93
Oil sardine	97
Pomfrets	87

Prawns	89
Rohu	97
Shark	93
Shrimp, small, dried	349
Sole	94
Surmai, fresh	92
Tengera, fresh	144
Meat & Poultry	
Beef	410
Duck	130
Egg, duck	181
Egg, hen	173
Goat meat (lean)	118
Liver, sheep	150
Mutton	194
Pigeon	137
Pork muscle	114
Snail, small	74
Turtle meat	86
Milk & Milk Products	
Buffalo milk	117
Cow milk	67
Goat milk	72
Human milk	65
Curds (yogurt), Cow milk	60
Butter milk	15
Skimmed milk	29
Cheese	348
Khoya of buffalo milk	421

Cow whole milk powder	496
Fats & Oils	
Butter	729
Ghee	900
Hydrogenated oil	900
Cooking oils (Groundnut, mustard, Coconut etc.)	900
Sugars	
Cane sugar	398
Honey	319
Sugar cane juice	300

In Europe and USA, all the manufacturers/packers of different foods are required to give the energy value and composition of those foods on the labels, by law. It is very easy for the consumer to know the amount of different constituents and their energy values.

Yogic Diet

Creative energy of food is 'Brahma'.

Nourishing energy of food is 'Vishnu'.

Spiritual energy of food is 'Shiva'.

After having understood the body requirements of different nutrients, I shall try to explain the diet which was recommended over 5000 years ago for people practising yoga.

Yogic diet is the diet, which is taken to keep the body and the mind pure so that it remains connected with the supreme energy. The main sources of energy to the body are:

(1) Sun energy
(2) Cosmic energy
(3) Food energy

A common individual derives his body energy from the sun and food where food plays a major role. Yogis with practice develop the ability to bring their basal metabolic rate down to a minimum. Yogis only eat to keep the body alive and healthy. In yoga a lot of importance is given to the state of the mind and it is said that the state of mind depends upon the sort of food one consumes.

In yoga, it is stated that depending upon the past deeds, the paternal deeds, which are transmitted to the human body through genes, an individual takes birth with a particular energy, in a particular environment, under particular circumstances, at a particular place, in a particular family. These energies, which are called *Gunas* and which comprise of primordial nature, are divided into three qualities. These correspond with matter, energy and consciousness and are given the names of Tamas (Matter), Rajas (Energy) and Sattava (Consciousness). Gunas have been described in detail in the chapter on evolution.

An individual is born with all the three Gunas but depending upon the factors explained earlier, a particular Guna dominates whereas the other two remain suppressed. All the three Gunas come to surface or dominance from time to time depending upon the circumstances.

People with Sattva dominance represent clear and pure mind, which in turn leads to self-realisation. Sattva also represent intelligence, harmony, peace and love. Sattvic people take only enough food, which is required for the survival of the body in optimum health. Hence, they prefer nourishing, simple natural foods, like fresh milk, fresh vegetables and fruits, natural nuts and natural cereals like wheat, maize, etc.

Yogic diet is a Sattvic diet. As mentioned earlier, the state of mind is very important to a yogi, hence it is important that the person who cooks food must be in a perfect stable state of mind and his whole mind should be engaged in the process of cooking at the time of cooking. It should be cooked with clean hands in clean and pure surroundings and absolutely clean utensils. Sattvic people also take care that the food is eaten with clean hands, with a calm and clean mind, thinking that this food is being offered to God. Every action of a Sattvic person is meditative. He puts his heart and soul into every act he performs and offers that act to God in a detached manner and accepts the results as a reward (Prasad).

People with Rajasic Guna dominating are born/ or acquire a turbulent mind. They always look outside to gratify their sensual desires. A mind agitated with desires is always an angry and manipulative mind, seeking power and fulfillment of the desires through fair or foul means. Rajasic qualities are action, turbulence, passion, aggression, competition, pain and strife. Rajasic people become mad for the possession of worldly gains and perform every act with a sense of attachment. To nourish these needs they love to eat foods, which tickle their palates, and give them pleasure and lots of energy (high in calories). These foods include various types of meat, milk products, cooked vegetables and fast foods.

People born with Tamas as the dominating Guna remain ignorant with a clouded mind in a state of sloth or sleep and lack concentration. The mind lacks activity and sensitivity and is dominated by subconscious forces. This state of mind is very near to the animal state of mind. Such people cannot discriminate between good and bad food, between fresh and stale food, between properly cooked and half cooked food, between nourishing and non-nourishing food and between a balanced and unbalanced diet and would eat any thing which comes their way.

A person practising yoga should try the following guidelines regarding eating habits so as to sustain a healthy body and a pure mind:

(1) He should eat only when he feels hungry.

(2) Pure food (organic) cooked at a clean place with good intentions should be eaten.

(3) With the first morsel of the food he should offer prayers to God and the entire food be considered as God-given gift (Prasad).

(4) Do not drink water while eating. Water should be taken half an hour (preferably one hour) after taking food.

(5) The food should be eaten with a calm mind concentrating on the eating process. The food should be neither cold nor hot.

(6) Do not indulge in talking while eating.

(7) The food should be chewed properly so that half of it is digested in the mouth. Too much spicy food is harmful for the mouth and the stomach.

(8) Salad and fruit should not be taken with the main meal, preferably these should be taken before the meal so as to fill part of the stomach. Milk which is thought to be a complete food should also be taken separately and it should replace a meal and not be in addition to the meal

(9) The selection of the food depends upon individual taste. The foods are selected out of sattvic diet (sattvic diet is mentioned in preceding paragraphs). Sattvic foods are usually low-calorie foods and should be mixed in such a way that it makes a balanced diet. Different varieties of food should not be mixed *e.g.* taking an acidic food with an alkaline food is not advisable.

(10) Stomach should never be completely filled with food. Enough space should be left for water and air, so as to provide enough space for the digestive processes.

(11) The mouth should be thoroughly rinsed after taking food

(12) A light walk for 15 to 20 minutes is recommended after taking food. A yogi performs Vjar asana after this, for a period of 15 to 20 minutes because it helps in the digestive process.

(13) The food which is taken should be earned and not begged.

(14) In yoga drinking ice cold water is not recommended. During summer fresh water should be drunk and during winter warm water is recommended. Yogis prefer to take warm water throughout the year, because it is thought that warm water taken frequently helps in keeping the digestive system clean.

Herbivorous versus Carnivorous

To be a vegetarian or a non-vegetarian has become a moral issue in modern times for spiritually/religiously enlightened people.

It is well known that in ancient times when there was no civilisation and food was scarce, humans survived and thrived on animal flesh. As a matter of fact animal flesh provides a perfect food for strength because it is rich in proteins, fat and vitamin B 12 (vitamin B 12 is essential for the formation of the blood), but it provides an inferior form of energy. The quality of energy provided by animal proteins is not as superior as that provided by carbohydrates like sugars, but the force of energy provided by animal flesh is much greater (hot, high in calories) which gives warmth and strength to the body by building the broken down tissues, whereas energy provided by vegetables, fruits (plants resources) and carbohydrates (sugars) is cool energy which is readily utilised by the brain and nervous tissue enhancing the process of imagination, intuition, observation and spirituality. That is why vegetarian food is thought to be a better source of energy.

Steroids and hormones which are fed to animals today make them produce more milk or increase their weight rapidly. But produce harmful effects in the human body if such animals/animal products are consumed by humans.

It is beyond doubt that animal food has its own place in the diet for certain sections of society, but vegetable food is recommended for people following the path of yoga, as it gives cool energy and directs the mind towards spirituality.

Intention, with which the food is plucked/bought, circumstances in which the food is prepared, environment in which the food is consumed, thought processes of the person at the time of consuming the food are all relevant to the body as well as the mind.

Visualisation of the animals being slaughtered for food, society/family tradition and various other factors influence one's choice to be a vegetarian or a non-vegetarian.

Fasting

Fasting is a process of cleansing the body by getting rid of all the bad energies. It implies depriving a particular system of its food *i.e.* seeing is a food for eyes, smelling is a food for the nose and thought is a food for the mind as bread, vegetables, fruits, etc. are food for the body.

Fasting enables a system to get rid of the bad and waste energy which is not required by the body, hence it should be thrown out. Fasting deprives the body of its daily requirements of food. Yoga recommends depriving different senses of their food at least once a week because it helps in calming down the nerves and increases the concentration of the mind.

Foods with a high oxalate content lead to formation of urinary stones

Palak, chaulai, tomatoes, cucumbers, amla, chickoo, cashew nut are rich in oxalates.

Foods rich in uric acid/purines can produce stone

Cauliflowers, brinjals (egg plant or aubergines), pumpkins, mushrooms are rich in uric acid.

Foods which are good and prevent the formation of urinary stones

Coconut Water: Contains dialysable bimolecular which stimulate demineralisation of the early phase of stone formation.

Corn: This is rich in Tartrates rates, which are good inhibitors of stone formation.

Barley: This acts as a diuretic, also rich in stone formation inhibitors.

Pineapple: Contains fibrins, which prevent stone formation. Pineapple is rich in dietary fiber, which reduces excretion of calcium in the urine.

Bananas: Are rich in Vitamin B6, which helps in breakdown of oxalic acid preventing stone formation.

Almonds: Are rich in magnesium and potassium, which act as stone formation inhibitors.

Lemons: Are rich in citric acid and prevent calcium oxalate stone formation.

Carrots: Are rich in plant acid, which inhibit stone formation. Carrots are also rich in Vitamin A. Lack of Vitamin A leads to urinary bladder stone formation.

Channa Dal: Inhibits stone formation.

Karela (Bitter Gourd): Contains magnesium phosphorus and phytoconstituents, which are helpful in preventing urinary stones and gout.

Yoga and Sex

6

YOGA AND SEX

After the survival instinct, sex comes next in the basic human instincts. Sexual union is essential for reproduction and propagation of species. Or else the species shall dwindle and cease to exist.

Before I embark upon a discussion regarding sexual energy and its yogic interpretation it is important to understand a few *terms*, which will be frequently used in this discussion.

(1) Love

Love is a soft, gentle, considerate, compassionate feeling created by the mind backed by an outpouring of energy, which takes the shape of the thought process, prevailing at that moment.

Love may be for God, parents, relatives or friends. You may be attached to them in a worldly sense but love itself is a completely detached feeling, that is why people find it difficult to express love in words. This feeling makes the body energy cool and you can experience it flowing through your eyes, tongue and actions.

(2) Orgasm

Orgasm is a very pleasant feeling, which not only relaxes the mind completely but also relaxes all the muscles of the body through the nerves. A person who experiences orgasm momentarily forgets everything, hence experiences only bliss (Ananda).

Orgasm is felt in the brain and is produced by the fulfillment of the desire of certain sensate foci. It is absolutely wrong to associate orgasm only with the sexual act, because one can achieve orgasm through visual sensations, by stimulation of some very sensitive areas in the body or even auditory orgasm can be enjoyed.

Usually sexual orgasm is associated with ejaculation in males. It is true that people experience orgasm at the time of ejaculation, but orgasm and ejaculation are two separate phenomena taking place at different levels. Ejaculation takes place at the physical level whereas orgasm takes place at the mental (brain) level, hence these two can be separated *i.e.* a person can get orgasm with external ejaculation. In "Eastern philosophy" orgasm and ejaculation are two separate phenomena, whereas in "Western philosophy" male orgasm without ejaculation is not possible.

(3) Internal Ejaculation

A person needs a lot of practice to ejaculate internally. A person can develop power either to take the semen upwards and ejaculate in the urinary bladder or ejaculate in the mind, but there is no external ejaculation. Here the internal ejaculation is synchronised with orgasm. Only few yogis are able to achieve this because of the hard work and patience involved.

(4) Brahamacharya

It is a wrong belief that Brahamacharya means abstinence from sex and preservation of energy.

Brahamacharya was based on the belief that loss of semen (Oja energy) was *'death'* and preservation of semen meant *'life'*.

In the true sense a Brahamachari is a person who has mastered the sacred scriptures *i.e. Vedas* and who sees divinity in all and everywhere. He is a perfect lover, having perfected the knowledge of Divine love.

A yogi trained in Brahamacharya has a store of vital energy, sharp intellect and can fight any injustice. Brahamacharya is another name for *wisdom*.

(5) Yoni

Female sexual and reproductive organs are called 'yoni' in Sanskrit. Yogis pray to *'yoni'* and meditate upon this because this is the place from where new energy (life) comes into existence.

During Roman times, all the roads in Europe used to lead to 'Rome'. Similarly in the body all the sensual energie's lead to *sexual energy*. Eyes love to see sexy things, ears love to hear sexy words/music, the tongue loves to taste/lick the sex, fingers love to play piano of sex and the nose goes mad after a sexy odour.

The body energy when converted to sexual energy becomes most powerful energy. The job of the yogi is to subdue sexual energy and change its direction so that it is converted into *spiritual energy*.

The source of the entire body energy is the same; it takes different forms for different acts. Ancient Hindus called it *Kundalini*, Chinese call it *Chi* and Taoists (ancient Chinese) called it *Yin & Yang*. The energy takes two different forms *i.e.* male and female. Human beings have both male and female characteristics. In males the male characteristics dominate, whereas in females the female characters dominate. In other words all of us have male as well as female energy.

According to Chinese belief "Taoism", the entire universe is composed of both male (Yang) and female (Yin) energy. A balance and harmony must be maintained between Yin and Yang and these energies should be exchanged frequently; this applies to sexual union as much as any other part of life.

Female Energy

In Indian mythology this is called *Shakti*. It is a crude form of energy involved with pattern, recognition, intuition, sensitivity and creative insight. All these are the functions of the right hemisphere of the brain. Hence right hemisphere of brain represents female energy and controls the left side of the physical body (each brain hemisphere controls the opposite side of the physical body). This is called crude energy because it is non-rational and is based on pure faith; logic has no place in it.

Male Energy

Indian mythology calls this energy *Shiva*. It is a refined form of energy responsible for rationalism, critical thinking and analytical sense. These are functions of the left hemisphere of the brain. Hence the left hemisphere represents male energy and controls the right side of the physical body.

When crude female energy and refined male energy unite, it produces refined and rational (logical) energy. Both these energies are of no use without each other, because 'Shakti' (female energy) is *Matter* and

'Shiva' (male energy) is *Mind,* when Matter meets Mind it comes alive and it is Matter which provides the residing place to the Mind. Without each other they have no value, but once they unite they become *Power.* Yoga teaches us to raise this power to perfection.

Yogis treat every act of life as worship. Every moment of a yogi is spent in worship and the act of sexual union was thought to be the highest form of worship. Hindus worship 'Shiva' (male energy) in the shape of 'Lingam' (phallus) in the 'Yoni' (female sexual organs), because it is from here the whole universe was created.

The sexual act is thought to be the most sacred act, where the union of two energies leads to the highest form of bliss, which is God. Before the act the energies are properly provoked by foreplay (caressing, kissing, fondling etc.) and they are regarded as Divine. Female energy being a crude form of energy takes longer to be provoked, once provoked it also takes longer to cool down.

During the act of sexual intercourse, there is not only exchange of physical energies, but also of spiritual energies. By exchanging energy you are acknowledging the true nature of the act, *i.e,* its divinity. It is not only an act of procreation but also of ultimate love.

In yoga the sexual act is used to increase, improve, expand and explore spirituality. Yoga recommends that both partners need to balance both the energies. No sex is as bad as unsatisfactory sex, because it is disharmonious. Sex should be used as a process of 'communication' with God.

A tremendous amount of energy is generated during sexual intercourse. Westerners believe that a sexual encounter must culminate in ejaculation to experience orgasm, whereas in yoga the focus is on multiple orgasms and not only on ejaculation. Yogis worship the sexual energy and during worship they enjoy the 'Bliss'.

During lovemaking and foreplay, male energy slowly works its way up the man's spine. Male energy is hotter and more volatile, hence it rises faster. It gets exhausted quickly, and lasts for a short period.

Female energy rises slowly upwards through the belly and breasts. Female energy is cooler, hence it rises slowly but is well sustained on the peak, women take longer to reach orgasm but are capable of enjoying multiple orgasms. Women take longer to be aroused and take longer to cool down. Here the 'Kundalani' energy acts as sexual energy. Depending upon the state of mind and relaxation of the two partners, some times there will be union of souls and some times not.

Sexual energy can take any of the following four forms:

(1) Orgasmic,

(2) Meditative,

(3) Spiritually enlightening and

(4) Combination of the above three forms.

Energy is transformed according to the need of the body, and not according to your expectation or desire. So your need is fulfilled at that particular time and you should go with it and not against it.

Yoga recommends sustaining sex for a longer period. The aim is to take the sensation higher and higher, till the male and female energies become one and there is a meeting of souls when both the partners go into a state of meditation and become one with the universe. Love is transformed to meditation; hence love and meditation become one.

In yoga it is said that in deep penetration love, meditation and God become one and that is Bliss.

In olden days, sexual union was only recommended for procreation and not for enjoyment. Enjoyment came as a part of the act. Research and evolution has proved that quality of genes improves with every act of ejaculation. In modern day and age sex has become an enjoyment because the world is saturated with human beings and procreation has lost its meaning. Sexual act is performed to satisfy our senses and to fulfill our basic human instinct. It is beyond doubt that sex has remained the most basic need of humans, ever since they came into existence and it will remain till our race will last. Sex has been exploited in the past and it will be exploited for times to come. Sex is being regularly enjoyed, because it has been observed that it keeps the individuals young in looks as well as in spirits. Just thinking about sex starts the flow of energy which in turn stimulates the production of sex hormones, their production reaches the peak during the act of sexual intercourse. These hormones give a feeling of well being and affect the skin, hair and other tissues of the body, rejuvenating them and imparting fresh and youthful looks to them.

Yoga and Sleep

7

Yoga and Sleep

Sleep is nature's process to allow the body to rest and re-energise. Normal sleep has two components *i.e.* light sleep and deep sleep. Light sleep pertains to 'rest', whereas deep sleep makes a person 'unconscious'. It is the deep sleep or unconsciousness, which forms a true part of sleep.

A yogi through the process of pranayam and meditation develops the abilities to go into deep sleep enjoying complete rest while remaining fully conscious. He goes into meditative sleep as soon as he puts his head on the pillow because his mind is absolutely blank and clear. He may get up from a bout of deep sleep after 1 or 2 hours fully conscious and absolutely refreshed.

A normal individual tries to sleep while his mind is full of thoughts. He goes into a phase of light sleep but his mind keeps on working and may go into a state of dreaming. When he gets up he feels tired, cannot concentrate and feels lost, because in the dream state the entire nervous system keeps on working because of the turbulent mind. Although the body of such a person lies static in bed his mind is neither stable nor peaceful.

Sleep can only be enjoyed and its advantages reaped when the mind is calm and preferably in the zero state. A peaceful mind gives peace to the body whereas a restless mind shatters the body.

With little practice a person practising yoga can control the mind to a reasonable extent. When he goes to sleep his mind is calm and enters the state of deep sleep fairly soon to reap its results.

Although *shavasana* has been described in the chapter on "Physical Rejuvenation" I think it will be appropriate to describe here the modified technique once again for a better understanding for complete relaxation of the body and the mind. The technique is divided into 5 stages:

Stage 1

This is a stage of *rest* in which the individual lies down on his back with his eyes closed, relaxing all parts of his body and takes long and deep breaths about 5 to 7 times a minute.

Stage 2

This is the stage of *inner observation*. In this stage the individual starts observing his breath, ultimately uniting his breath with his mind. This union of breath and mind creates tremendous amount of energy, which is taken into different parts of the body through the mind's gaze, so as to rejuvenate those parts. Special attention is paid to those particular parts/ points, which are either diseased or weak so that those parts are fully energised and a positive thought that this energy is acting as a heeling force for those particular parts brings the desired results.

All body parts feel completely relaxed and energised during this stage.

Stage 3

In this stage the individual meditates on the chakras. For better understanding of chakras, the reader is referred to the chapter on "Yoga Energy System". In this stage one also meditates on the five elements of the body.

- By concentrating on the Muladhara Chakra, one meditates on the *Earth* element and feels the heaviness in the bones, muscles, skin and arteries etc.
- By concentrating on Svadhishthana Chakra, one meditates on *Water* element of the body and visualises the blood flowing through one's body and a cool flowing taste in the mouth.
- By concentrating on Manipura Chakra, one meditates on the *Fire* element of the body. One can visualise the energy running in all parts of body through the energy channels (nadis)
- By concentrating on Anahat Chakra, one meditates on *Air* element of the body and feels coolness and love throughout the body.
- By concexntrating on Vishuddha Chakra, one meditates on the *cosmic* energies by the process of visualisation and purification of the energy body.

Stage 4

This is the stage of super consciousness or divinity. In this stage after having meditated on five elements of the body, one directs one's breath and mind towards "Ajna Chakra" where he tries to gain the highest knowledge and ultimately directs his meditative attention towards "Sahasrara Chakra" for attainment of universality and bliss.

Stage 5

After having gone through the meditative stages, one reverts to observing one's breath. Keeping the mind with the breath, he starts "Japa meditation" *i.e.* chanting of a mantra or a name pertaining to any religion one believe in, and try to lose the mind in the rhythm of that mantra.

Yogic Sleep

A person practising yoga trains his mind to remain in a relaxed state under all circumstances. Yogic sleep is different from deep sleep, because in yogic sleep a person goes into deep sleep but remains fully conscious.

A yogi can sleep any where at any time to relax his body and mind. He needs far less sleep than an ordinary person to rejuvenate his body.

Advantages of yogic sleep

The advantages of yogic sleep are:

(1) It makes the mind sharp.
(2) It helps in healing the physical body.
(3) It cures tension, heart disease, high blood pressure and psychiatric illnesses.
(4) It helps in coordination of different systems of the body.
(5) It takes away body fatigue.
(6) It helps in understanding the real self.
(7) It purifies the body energy.

Yoga and Prayer

8

Yoga and Prayer

Prayer is a process by which a person can give vent to his feelings, release his tension, direct his mind to a particular direction, unite the body energies and give them a direction. One always prays to the Supreme.

What does prayer do?

(1) It makes a person humble.

(2) It allows one to shed his ego.

(3) It makes a person fearless.

(4) It calms down the body energies and purifies them.

(5) It calms down the mind; hence the mind develops the power to analyse.

(6) Prayer helps in conversion of the ordinary body energy/ sex energy into spiritual energy.

(7) Prayer subdues hatred, attachments, anger and greed, hence makes a person submissive.

(8) Prayer acts as an outlet of one's emotions.

When and where to pray?

One can pray anywhere, at any time, in any posture. It is a feeling, which usually starts from the heart (Anahata Chakra). A yogic prayer involves the entire body energy. It starts from the *Muladhara chakra,* travels upwards through *Svadhishthana, Manipura chakras* and is concentrated in the *Anahata chakra*. From here it moves up to *Vishuddha chakra* where it is purified moves up further to have a soothing effect at the *Ajna chakra* and unites with the Cosmos through the *Sahasrara chakra*.

What is the purpose of prayer?

The main purpose of prayer is to unite the individual body energy to the universal cosmic energy to find solution/ answers to daily situations, whether these are personal, involving a community, a country or the world at large.

How to pray?

Prayer may be said silently by concentrating at the level of the Heart chakra or may be performed loudly with the help of the Vishuddha chakra. Group/ community prayers are usually performed with a loud voice/chanting, which helps in awakening the dormant energies.

A silent prayer has more emotions attached to it but a prayer is a prayer whether performed silently or loudly. It gives the same bliss/ananda to the performer. Ultimately it is the peace of mind which matters.

A prayer, which involves all the energy of the body and is said with a pure heart, is always answered. When I say answered I mean you are always guided by your higher self.

Importance of prayer has been mentioned in the Vedas. Vedas recommend Gayatri mantra as a prayer for the benefit of the whole universe.

Gayatri Mantra

"Om, Bhur, Bhuvah, Swah
That, Savitur, Varenyam
Bhargo Devasya Dhiemahi
Dhiyo, YoNah, Parchodayat."

This means:

"Oh, Lord of the Lords, bestower of life, purity and bliss.

Omnipresent and omniscient, creator of the entire universe, we meditate on your divine wisdom and ask for the pardon of our sins and request you to enlighten our intellects.

We pray to the almighty and ask for his guidance.

Our intellect should never be deprived of your radiance and your radiance may ever shine on our intellect and inspire us to do good deeds and follow the path of righteousness."

Yoga and Death

9

YOGA AND DEATH

Every creation must end one day. It is the matter which disintegrates, decays or dissolves, this process of dissolution is called *Death*. It is the law of the Nature. It is matter which dies or disintegrates, energy never dies, it changes shape.

Human body is created by the union of male and female energies which dwell in matter called body which is basically made of four elements *i.e.* Earth, Water, Fire and Air. All these elements are kept in balance and equilibrium and are given a shape which becomes a human body. When energy is infused into it from cosmos, it becomes a human being. Both matter as well as energy grow and expand slowly till they reach a peak and then the decline starts till the matter disintegrates into its basic elements and energy is liberated which takes a different shape.

Human body needs proper systems for its functioning and growth. The matter takes the shape of specialised cells to form these systems. The whole body is controlled by a super system called the nervous system.

A cell is the smallest unit of a system which is capable of independent survival *i.e.* it has matter as well as energy, it also contains memory of past lives/existence stored in DNA (Deoxyribonucleic Acid) present in the genes of its nucleus. A group of cells makes a tissue which is capable of performing specialised functions. A group of tissues makes a system. Systems which assimilate/imbibe energy are Respiratory System, Digestive System, Circulatory System etc. Systems like the Excretory System throw out the waste/bad energy from the body. Some tissues/systems perform the dual function of taking in the good energy and throwing out the bad energy like Skin, Digestive and Respiratory Systems. All these Systems are controlled by a Super System which is capable of transmitting as well as firing the energy. This System as mentioned before is called the Nervous System.

Every cell has a life span after which it disintegrates and is replaced by a new cell which carries the memory of the old cell. At the time of dissolution energy leaves the cell and the cell disintegrates into its basic elements which go and combine with the elements of the nature.

Human body is composed of billions of such cells which degenerate/regenerate thousand of times, till the whole body disintegrates or dies. This phenomenon is called Death.

Hence at the time of death, the energy leaves the body and the cells disintegrate into basic elements. This energy has been called Atma in Hindu philosophy. It enters another matter and gives life to it, carrying the memory of its past actions/deeds with it in its DNA and this was named Reincarnation in Hindu philosophy. According to this philosophy, this process goes on till the energy is purified to its extreme. This absolute pure energy goes and combines with the

Universal Cosmic Energy. Hence this process of life and death goes on and on.

Death can also take place if the supply of Vital Energy is suddenly stopped to the body, it is like switching off the light, as happens in Asphyxia. Here the energy to the cells is suddenly cut off and they stop functioning instantaneously because of shock.

If the energy supply to the body gets low and remains low, as happens in starvation or chronic anemia, the cells try to adjust but die a slow death as happens in Cachexia. In such cases the cells die a gradual death.

Once the individual dies, the body goes through the process of disintegration and is converted into its basic elements: the Air gets back to the atmospheric air, Fire gradually subsides and dwindles away, the Water evaporates and the Earth goes back to the earth.

A true yogi is the one who lives his life the yoga way following all its principles from an early age. Since his mind learns to get detached from the senses and becomes single pointed by the process of meditation, he learns to control the supply of the energy to the body. He also trains his body cells to survive and function at minimum energy levels. In extreme cases he gets so much control over his energy that he can die by his own Will when the purpose of his being born is fulfilled. Hence a true yogi can control his death. When he dies of his own Will he is known to attain Samadhi or Nirvana, which means that he can get out of the cycle of birth and death, his soul which is nothing but energy rises up and joins the Universal Cosmic Energy.

The death should always be rejoiced and not mourned because it completes a cycle and the person gets ready to be born again depending on his Karmas.

In Kali

is agai

human

(a

(b

(c)

(d

Thi

one

individu

an anim

whole

eating

"total

The

whole

transfo

(a)

CONCLUSION

In Kali Yuga we are striving to satisfy our senses, which is against the nature of our soul. The final goal of the human race is:

(a) To identify with the soul, which is a part of universal cosmic energy.

(b) To find the relationship of the soul with the body.

(c) To find the functions of the soul.

(d) To find ways and means by which an individual soul can find union with its Mother Energy (Universal Cosmic Energy), after having fulfilled its purpose.

The universe and man are one indivisible existence, one "total whole". Anything that appears to us as an individual entity, whether it is a planet, man, atom or an animal is a temporary manifestation of the "total whole". Every activity whether it is birth or death, eating or loving is a temporary manifestation of the "total whole".

Each one of us is but a cell in the body of this "total whole". This cell performs its function and passes away, transformed into another manifestation.

The aspirants of yoga should engage themselves in:

(a) Selfless service for self-purification.

(b) Lead a disciplined life with principles and goals.

(c) Indulge in intense, regular and systematic practice of yoga principles.

(d) Should enjoy sex as meditation

(e) Should not be attached to sense objects.

(f) Every act should be done with a detached mind and as an offering to God.

This whole unrest in the world has been created by us because we do not listen to the voice of our soul. Once we go back to the path of spirituality, we shall start enjoying our lives. We have forgotten that we came empty-handed and shall leave empty-handed. What we perform is all jugglery. We take with us only our good or bad karmas.

Yoga and its principles have gone through an evolution in the last fifty years. Individuals as well as organisations have exploited yoga commercially for their monetary gains. It is not yoga as a whole which has been exploited, but it has been exploited in bits and pieces. Mostly the Physical Rejuvenation, Pranayam and Meditation have been exploited. Different organisations and so-called yogis have tried to give their own names to these parts of yoga and made money out of it.

Yoga in toto was promoted by Gurukul in India. This organisation opened residential centres where students were taught yogic way of life and made to lead their lives on the basis of yoga principles.

In my own experience yoga is more prevention than cure. Keeping the nerves calm by pranayam can definitely contribute to alleviation of symptoms to an extent but it does not last long, if the person is not motivated enough to make pranayam as a part of his normal routine in daily life.

Bibliography

Abhedananda Swami, *Yoga Psychology*, Ram Krishna Vedanta Math, Calcutta, India.

Andrews Ted, *How to develop and use Psychic Touch*, Llewellyn Publications, St. Paul, Minnesota, U.S.A.

Aurobindo Sir, *The Supramental Manifestation*.

Austin James H.M.D, *Zen & the Brain*, MIT Press Cambridge, U.K.

Avalon Arthur, *The Serpent Power*, Dover Publications, New York, U.S.A.

Baker Douglar, *The Techniques of Astral Projections*, Baker Publications, U.K.

Bakhru H.K., *Herbs that Heal*, Orient Paperbacks, New Delhi, India.

Bartlett Sarah, *Auras and How to Read Them*, Collins and Brown Ltd., London, U.K.

Bentov Itzhak, *Stalking the Wild Pendulum*, Destiny Books, Rochester, Vermont, U.S.A.

Buess Lyn, *Numerology in the New Age*, Light Technology, Sedona U.S.A.

Buzan Tony, *Use Your Head*, B.B.C., London, U.K.

Chandappa Rohan, *The Little Book of Stress*, Ebury Press, London.

Charak K.S., *Surya, The Sun God*, Uma Publications, New Delhi, India.

Chinmayananda Swami, *Meditation & Life*, Chinmaya Nanda Mission, Mumbai, India.

Chinmayananda Swami, *Kaivalya Upanishad*, Central Chinmaya Mission Trust, Mumbai, India.

Chinmayananda Swami, *Kath Upanishad*, Central Chinmaya Mission Trust, Mumbai, India.

Choa Kok Sui Master, *Miracles through Pranic Healing*, Institute of Inver Studies, Philippines.

Craze Richard, *Tantric Sexuality*, Hodder and Stoughton, London.

Dalrymple William, *The Age of Kali*, Flamingo (a division of Harper Collins), New York, London.

Frawley David, *Ayurvedic Healing*, Motilal Banarsidass, Delhi, India.

Gawain Shakti, *Creative Visualization*, Full Circle, New Delhi, India.

Gawain Shakti, *Meditation*, Full Circle, New Delhi, India.

Gokhle Namita, *The Book of Shiva*, Penguin Books, New Delhi.

Gopalan C., Sashtri B.V. Rama, Balasubramanian S.C., *Nutritive Value of Indian Foods*, Indian Council of Medical Research, Hyderabad, India.

Greogory P. Fields, *Religion Therapeutics*, Motilal Banarasidas, Delhi, India.

Grewal Rohina, *The Book of Ganesha*, Penguin Books, New Delhi.

Hillman James, *The Soul's Code*, Bantam Books, London, U.K.

Janet Balaskas, *Preparing for Birth with Yoga*, Shaftesbury, U.K.

Judith Anodea, *Eastern Body, Western Mind*, Celestial Arts, Berkeley, U.S.A.

Judith Anodea, *Wheels of Life*, Liewellya Publications, St. Paul, Minnesota, U.S.A.

Kavl Jankinath, *Bhavani Nama Sahasra Stutih*, Ram Krishna Ashram Siri Nagar, India .

Krupp P.G., *Drugless Therapy*, Ocean Books Pvt. Ltd., New Delhi, India.

Levin Michael, *Spiritual Intelligence*, Hodden and Stroughton, London, U.K.

Levin Michael, *Path to Deepest Self*, Dorling Kindersley Ltd., London, U.K

Low Jennifer and Danino Michel, *The Mind of the Cells*, Institute of de Recherches Evolutives, Paris, France.

Macritchie James, *The Chi Kung Way*, Harper Collins, San Franscisco, U.S.A.

Marshall, Lyn, *Wake up to Yoga*, Ward Lock Ltd., London, U.K.

Melchizedek Drunvalo, *The Ancient Secret of the Flower of Life*, Vols I & II, Light Technology Trust, U.S.A.

Mookerjee Ajit, *Kundalini*, Thames & Hudson Ltd., London, U.K.

Moore Thomas, *The Planets Within*, Lindisfarne Press, Hudson, New York, U.S.A.

Moss Robert, *Dream Gates*, Three Rivers Press, New York, U.S.A.

Muktananda Swami, *Chit Shakti Vilas*, Ram Krishna Math, Calcutta, India.

Myss Caroline, *Sacred Contracts*, Bantam Books, London, U.K.

Naparstek Belleruth, *Your Sixth Sense*, Harper Collins, San Franscisco, USA.

Orloff Judith, *Intuitive Healing*, Rider, London, U.K.

OSHO, *Book of Secrets*.

Paramhansa Yogananda, *Autobiography of a Yogi*.

Parmananda Swami, *Vedanta in Practice*.

Peat David F, *Synchronicity*, Bantam Books, New York, U.S.A.

Peter J. D'Adams, *Eat Right for Your Type*, Century, London, U.K.

Prabhupada Swami, *The Perfection of Yoga*, The Bhakti Vedanta Book Trust, London, U.K.

Radha Krishana, *Translation of Gita*.

Reiter Russel J, *Melatonin*, Bantam Books, New York, U.S.A.

Roy Bikek Deb and Roy Dipali Deb, *Atharva Veda, Yajur Veda, Rig Veda*, Books For All, Delhi, India.

Sagan Samuel, M.D, *Awakening the Third Eye*, Clair Vision, Australia.

Sankracharya, *Eight Upanishads*, Advaita Ashram, Calcultta, India.

Sharma G.C., *Brihat Parasara Hora Shashtra*, Sagar, New Delhi, India.

Shepard Leslie, *Living With Kundalini*, Shambhla, Boston (U.S.A.), London (U.K.).

Shivananda Yoga Center, *The Book of Yoga*, Ebury Press, London, U.K.

Sivananda Swami, *Kundlini Yoga*, Yogananda Vedanta Forest Academy, Rishikesh, U.P., India.

Siddhapeeth Gurudev, Ganesh Puri, Maharashtra, India.

Tolle Eckhart, *The Power of Now*, Yogi Impressions, Mumbai, India.

Varenne Jean, *Yoga & Hindu Tradition*, University of Chicago Press, London, U.K.

Verma Pavan K., *The Book of Krishna*, Penguin Books, New Delhi.

Worldwood Valirie Anu, *Fragmented Mind*.

Yoga, Asnas, Pranayama, Mudras, Kiryas, Vivekanand Kendra, Chennai, India.

Zukav Gary, *The Seat of the Soul*, The Random House Group, London, U.K.

INDEX